GRACE, FOOD, AND EVERYTHING IN BETWEEN

Discover the transforming power of grace to set you free from food and body shame.

Aubrey Golbek, MS, RDN

GRACE, FOOD, AND EVERYTHING IN BETWEEN

www.gracefueled.com
First Printing: 2018
Fonts Used: Garamond, Lemon Tuesday, League Gothic, Avenir Next
Cover Design By: Jeff Hertzler

Scripture, unless otherwise noted, is taken from The Holy Bible, English Standard Version, Copyright © 2001 by Crossway, a publishing ministry of Good News Publishers.

Scripture quotations marked TPT are from The Passion Translation®. Copyright © 2017, 2018 by Passion & Fire Ministries, Inc. Used by permission. All rights reserved. ThePassionTranslation.com.

Scripture quotations marked (NIV) are taken from the Holy Bible, New International Version®, NIV®. Copyright © 1973, 1978, 1984, 2011 by Biblica, Inc.™ Used by permission of Zondervan. All rights reserved worldwide. www.zondervan.com The "NIV" and "New International Version" are trademarks registered in the United States Patent and Trademark Office by Biblica, Inc.™

This content is the sole expression and opinion of its author, designed to provide information and motivation to its readers. This book is not intended as a substitute for the medical advice of physicians. The reader should regularly consult a physician in matters related to his/her health and particularly to any symptoms that may require diagnosis or medical attention.

The author shall not be liable for any physical, psychological, emotional, financial, or commercial damages, including but not limited to, special, incidental, consequential or other damages.

The names of clients and friends in this book have been changed to protect the privacy of the individuals mentioned.

Any internet addresses (websites, blogs, social media accounts), books or podcasts in this book are offered as a resource. They are not intended in any way to imply or be an endorsement by the author. The author does not vouch for the contents of these items or addresses for the life of this book.

ISBN: 9781728623061

To all those

in bondage, to the ones who've given up on breaking free on their own, may you find the one who can set you free forever:

"Now the Lord is the spirit, and where the spirit of the Lord is, there is freedom."

2 Corinthians 3:17 NIV

Praise for Grace, Food, and Everything in Between

Grace, Food, and Everything in Between is an easy read with a powerful message. Aubrey writes from the perspective of a friendly, but professional dietitian, sharing her personal struggles with food and victories in the Lord that both educate, inspire, and relieve the pressure surrounding the endless debate of "what's right" to eat for each person.

I walked away from reading each chapter with a renewed mind, enabling me to consume my next meal with joy and without the endless choices consuming my thoughts. I no longer felt like I had to give an excuse for what I was eating because the advice she offers throughout is not only practical but grounded in the gospel.

Thanks to *Grace, Food, and Everything in Between*, I feel free to eat my favorite candy out in the open without binging, empowered to wisely choose food that nourishes me in body and soul, and enjoy food as a gift from the Lord, instead of using it as an ensnaring coping mechanism. I highly recommend this book to anyone who wants to break away from the internal accusations of our diet culture and be filled with the nourishment of grace-based eating.

Kasey B. Shuller

Author of *Rest and Rise*
and *Love Beyond Looks*

TABLE OF CONTENTS

Introduction

THIS ONE'S FOR YOU

Maybe you're reading this page and you're thinking, oh joy, another book about eating—is it going to make a difference? Maybe you're unsure whether you even want to start it; you could be wondering whether it'll be helpful, or like the rest of the books on food and health, it'll end up collecting dust on the abandoned bookshelf in your garage.

In the interest of saving you time and money, and also encouraging you to read further, let me preface by telling you who this book IS for. This book is for all those who are stuck in a cycle of shame, dieting, and low self-worth. It's for my fellow control freaks and perfectionists who can't seem to let go of the reigns on their life and entrust them to God. It's for those in bondage to a barrage of food and body image concerns. It's for the well-intending people saying, "I just want to know how to eat healthfully." But mostly, it's for the people who, like me, are sick of striving for worthiness and are in need of the overwhelming, all-encompassing, good news of grace.

If you nodded your head to any of that, if you're burnt out on religion and you've also struggled with food or exercise at some point, then this book is for you. By all means, read on, and welcome. Believers and skeptics alike are welcome; I'm not picky with who I blabber on to (ask my husband). I'm just happy you're here.

First, introductions are in order. My name is Aubrey, I'm a former slave to people pleasing, control, food, and exercise. But, by the grace of God, and grace alone, I've been set free from all of that. Now, it's my mission as a registered dietitian and friend of Jesus, to implore, encourage, and equip people with the same truths that set me and so many others free. And over the next 220 pages, I hope to do just that for you!

Before I go on, be warned: this message of grace I'm sharing hasn't changed in over 2,000 years. What I write is not new, it's not brain science either, but that doesn't make it any less radical. Pure, unadulterated grace is all-consuming, makes zero sense to our natural mind, and is powerful enough to accomplish all things.

As you might have guessed, my encounter with grace involves a struggle with food, perfectionism, and worthiness. Not coincidentally, I spent a lot of time and money going to school to become a registered dietitian nutritionist. This book is the result of my encounter with grace and subsequent freedom with food, and a whole bunch of other things. It has a lot to do with healing our relationship to food, but more to do with our relationship with the one who made us and calls us a worthy and beloved friend.

The chapters to come are full of stories from my own life and those of my clients, friends, and family. They're sprinkled with a little self-deprecating humor, seasoned heavily with scripture, and doubly marinated in the gospel of grace.

The first half of the book encompasses the foundational truths we must understand and cling to in order to take hold of freedom from food, exercise, and body image concerns. I wholeheartedly believe, and Romans 12:2 confirms, that we are transformed, not by practical behavior management, but by the renewing of our minds and the alignment of our beliefs with the word of God. That's why I've chosen to lay out a foundation of grace before I ever give practical tips.

The second half of this book is chalk full of practical applications for eating and living free from diets, food worries, and body preoccupation. I draw from scripture, my education and experience as a dietitian, and the latest scientific research on intuitive eating to give you guidelines for becoming a normal, free eater.

At the end of each chapter, you'll find reflection questions. These are designed to help you digest, absorb, and utilize the content from each chapter. Of course, these questions would be great if discussed in a small group setting. So, if you're up for it, grab a couple friends and go through the book together. Grace isn't new, but it's pretty countercultural, especially when it comes to food, so the more friends you bring along with you on this journey, the less likely you'll stumble along the way.

What follows is an honest outpouring of my heart. Through my imperfect words, I pray that the perfect God of love and truth that raised a man, Jesus, from the dead 2,000 years ago and set the captives free will reveal grace to you afresh. I pray that you'll leave this book changed and freed, not by the power of my words, but by the transforming power of the King of the universe, the lover of your soul. I pray that you'll leave with a health that permeates from your spirit to your soul, your body, and every other aspect of your life.

Let me tell you, those are some lofty prayers y'all. But I'm believing for them anyway! With that in mind, go grab yourself a cup of joe, or in my case a chocolate chip cookie, and let's dig into the nitty gritty of grace, food, and everything in between.

Chapter 1

THE INSIDIOUS SIDE OF WELLNESS CULTURE

"For freedom Christ has set us free; stand firm therefore, and do not submit again to a yoke of slavery."

GALATIANS 5:1 ESV

WELLNESS CULTURE AND THE NOT SO "WELL" RESULTS

In a time where restaurants selling smoothie bowls are springing up all over the place and companies offering onsite fitness facilities and standing desks are landing the best employees, wellness has never been more popular. We live in a wellness culture. We praise people for focusing on healthy eating and exercise, and we glorify social media influencers who alternate sharing photos of their latest super food meal with shots of their perfectly toned bodies as they attend the latest trendy fitness class. We hold these people on a pedestal and try our darndest to measure up, but where has it gotten us?

For a majority of Americans, wellness culture has given us a preoccupation with food, exercise, and our body. At best this means we worry about food and exercise several times a day and feel guilty when we "slip up." At worst, we're completely consumed by food and exercise thoughts, obsessed with our own appearance and fitness, an obsession which leaves little time or energy for family, friends, or anything else worthwhile. The wellness obsession becomes a form of bondage, one that's socially acceptable, and even encouraged.

Women are particularly susceptible to this sort of bondage. According to a survey conducted of 4,000 U.S. women by SELF-magazine, 65-75% of women suffer from disordered eating. [1] Disordered eating comes into play when we regularly hold onto harmful and inaccurate beliefs about food and our bodies, resulting in unhealthy eating behaviors that interfere with the quality of our daily life. What's more, 20 million U.S. women (and 10 million men) will develop a full-blown eating disorder within their lifetime. [2,3] What all of these souls have in common is a culture that places worth and social standing in physical appearance. How are they told to improve their appearance and worth? They're told to lose weight through clean eating, an ambiguous term at best, and exercise.

The pursuit of wholeness or value from weight loss, or even physical wellness, by means of healthy eating and exercise, may seem harmless, and even beneficial on the surface, but the pursuit of worth from anything other than the cross of Jesus Christ is a sneaky form of slavery. In Galatians 5:1, Paul urges Christians: it is "for freedom Christ has set us free; stand firm therefore, and do not submit again to a yoke of slavery." By trusting physical wellness for our wholeness, we're effectively submitting to a yoke of bondage again.

Believers are not immune to being oppressed by the bondage of food and body image obsession. I've met many people with anorexia nervosa, a life-threatening eating disorder. A large portion of those individuals were professing Christians. Each person told stories of unknowingly submitting themselves to slavery in the name of good behavior and "taking better care of their bodies."

There is no question about the impact of wellness culture on the church; it's not uncommon to hear leaders preaching and encouraging church members to focus on restricting certain "bad" foods and burning calories in the gym to achieve health. The insidious side of this well-intended message is people attaching their hope and morality to eating, whether they realize it or not. It's a sneaky, slippery slope from labeling food as good or bad to labeling ourselves good or bad for eating the food. This self-inflicted judgment results in feelings of shame and condemnation over something as simple and necessary as eating.

THE DIET SHAME CYCLE

I've seen it too many times: sometimes it starts out of fear of death and disease and other times it's out of intentions to live an effective joyful life; we decide to "get healthy." Whatever the reason, we're usually told to lose weight, eat better, and exercise more. So, we do what seems logical: we go on a diet. We stop eating sugar, fat, or gluten and start exercising harder and longer. Usually the first time we diet we see quick results with weight loss. The weight loss and the attention that comes with it garner positive attention from other people. It feels good; it can even be described as intoxicating.

Flash-forward a few weeks, months, maybe even a year later: those of us who've dieted eventually get tired of restricting food and forcing exercise. We fall back into old patterns and even begin bingeing on previously off-limit foods, feeling terrible and helpless. Convinced that the problem is our broken body or lack of self-control, we might try a new diet, this time with more "resolve". But the mindset and beliefs haven't changed, so the outcome is the same. The cycle continues. With each successive weight loss attempt, dieters erode trust in their bodies and lose self-confidence. Weight loss becomes the primary goal, and the point on which everything else in life hinges, including identity.

As you can see, what starts out as an attempt to get healthy can quickly turn into a lifelong battle with weight, resulting in shame, stress, lack of self-esteem, and often, poorer health outcomes.

At this point you're probably wondering what in the world we're supposed to do about the rising rates of cardiovascular disease, diabetes, and other chronic illnesses if it's not losing weight or buckling down on healthy eating and exercise.

I understand your concern. After all, we've been told over and over again that weight loss is the key to health. We've been fed sneaky messages that tell us how we eat and exercise are a reflection of our worth as human beings. This is a lie from the enemy. Before we can address the health of our bodies, we must dismantle this false belief and replace it with truth. The truth is our worth is inherent. We were created by a God who loves us so much that he sent his only son, Jesus, to die for us while we were still imperfect sinners. We didn't earn this sacrifice. He did it because He loves and values us as we are. Our worth then, has nothing to do with our healthy behaviors, how we look, what we do for a living, or how successful we are. Our worth is already established.

When we start with this truth in mind we can begin to address our physical health from a grace-fueled perspective. This starts with believing that God has freely forgiven our imperfections and supplies us with His extravagant, unlimited love and favor, despite us doing nothing to earn or keep it. From this radical belief we're able to transform our mindset, followed by our emotions and desires, and finally our behaviors. But we must remember, Jesus is in the business of total transformation, not external behavior change. His grace is sufficient to make over every area of our lives, which certainly includes our health and actions.

IT'S TIME FOR A NEW THOUGHT

The majority of diets and books on health are aimed at changing behaviors, but what these programs lack is the necessary thought shift that always precedes permanent behavior change. In Romans 12:2 (NIV), Paul writes, "Do not conform to the pattern of this world but be transformed by the renewing of your mind. Then you will be able to test and approve what God's will is—His good, pleasing and perfect will." In the same way, we are called to renew our mindset on food and exercise and align our beliefs with God's Word, not with the beliefs of the world. Then, our relationship with food can be transformed to give Him glory.

The pattern of this world for eating and health is flawed. If diets and obsession with clean eating, exercise, and body weight were helpful, they would have worked by now! We wouldn't have people stuck in a never-ending cycle of dieting and body hate. It's time to be transformed by a new thought, a thought rooted in grace and truth.

This book will point you to the truth found in scripture concerning food, our bodies, identity, and worth; explore what the scientific research actually says about eating, dieting, and weight loss; and systematically lay the foundation of grace we have in Christ to live an abundant life, free from food and body image obsession.

As I write this, I'm deeply humbled by the transformation God has done in my own heart concerning food and body image. He's taken me from obsessed, self-righteous, and full of anxiety to at peace, energized, and full of joy. Better yet, He's allowed me to witness other sweet souls transformed by a grace-fueled mindset on health.

As you embark on this journey to end the dieting-shame cycle, and finally find rest in your relationship with food and your body, know that I am praying for each one of you. May your mind be opened to the truth; may God speak through these words. May He set you free from everything that hinders you. I know that as you trust God to renew your mind, He will be faithful to complete every good work He is starting in you!

REFLECTION QUESTIONS:

1. How has wellness culture affected your beliefs about your worth and identity?

2. What does God's grace mean to you? Are you trying to earn approval or worth through anything other than God's grace?

3. What diets have you been on? What inspired you to go on that first diet? In the long run, 6-12 months or 2 years later, did that diet help you feel better around food?

4. What concerns about food, exercise, or body image have held you back from God's calling in your life? What specific steps can you take to start living your calling as you are?

Chapter 2

NOURISH YOUR SOUL FIRST

"Beloved, I pray that all may go well with you and that you
may be in good health, as it goes well with your soul."

3 JOHN 1:2 ESV

SOUL & BODY HEALTH GO HAND-IN-HAND

When I was a swimmer, my coaches used to urge my
teammates and me to visualize our races. They asked us to
imagine everything from the rate of our arms as they sliced
through water and the feeling of our legs as they kicked up
waves, to the best time we'd inevitably see displayed on the
timeclock at the finish. If I'm being honest, at the time I
thought all of this was just a little "woo-woo." But as the
years have passed, I've discovered the wisdom in those
visualization sessions.

The truth is that what we think, believe, and meditate
on directly affects our emotions, actions, and physical health.
Research reveals that our thoughts and imaginings have
physical consequences. For example, when an athlete
imagines himself shooting the perfect free throw over and

over again, the motor complex associated with that movement fires up and prepares his muscles to act, even while he remains seated and unmoving. Further, repetitive visualization of this action may enable his body to shoot more effectively when game time rolls around.[1]

On the downside, we know that mental stress, caused by things like time pressure or anger can cause negative consequences in the body. When it comes to digestion, when the brain senses stress it signals to our gut's nervous system to stop or slow down its work, diverting the gut's blood flow and energy to the rest of the body while releasing stress hormones that prepare us for action. Over time, the presence of food in the gut without adequate support from the body for digestion may result in sensitivities and bacterial imbalances.[2] Additionally, if mental stress continually hogs all of our bodies' resources, our digestive system will object by sending loud and uncomfortable signals to the brain that something is wrong. This may be related to the onset of increased gut sensitivity conditions such as Irritable Bowel Syndrome.[2]

Clearly, our thoughts and imaginings, and the way we respond to stressors, have the power to produce positive and negative outcomes in our physical bodies. The Apostle John understood this. He understood that soul health, which is mental and emotional well-being, was related to physical health when he wrote his third letter to the early Christian Church. He greeted them by letting them know that he was praying for them to prosper in their physical health just as, or to the same degree, their soul was prospering in Christ (3 John 1:2). And just as John prayed for the believers to experience physical health AND soul health, God also wants us to experience both. However, our heavenly father is focused on our hearts first and foremost. As such, He works by healing all three parts of us: spirit, soul, and body. I do not believe He is in the business of healing bodies at the expense of our relationship with Him, or our soul's inner peace. That is the world's way of healing, not His.

Grace fueled health involves meeting our souls' needs first. It means cultivating a peaceful heart and a relaxed mind. In God's kingdom we learn to nourish our inner person first, until we're completely full and satisfied, content in who we are and who we are created to be. This kind of health results in a deep confidence and appreciation for life.

If you've ever met a truly confident person, you know just how amazing it is to find someone who loves life and isn't swayed by storms or seasons. I'm not talking about bravado or fake confidence, the type that seeks out attention and affirmation as a salve for our own wounds and insecurities. I'm talking about real confidence, the kind that results in walking through life intentionally, not running frantically after meaning, but striding steadily into one's purpose.

None of us are perfect, but I have met a few people with that sort of confidence—it's an attractive quality. Every person in my life who had that confidence has also been a believer. Just like these individuals, God wants our contentedness in Him to set us apart from the rest of the world; He wants it to draw others in so that we have more opportunities to share the reason for the hope that we have.

From a physical health perspective, being confident in whose you are, and content in who God created you to be, makes it ten times more likely that you'll want to take care of your body—a completely made up statistic, but you get the point. Logically speaking, if we are unhappy with the person that we are, if we feel unworthy and unlovable, why would we act to nurture and care for our physical bodies? Instead, those of us who are unfulfilled and disquieted in our soul tend to relate to food and health in one of three ways:

- One, we use restrictive eating, exercise, and the pursuit of "perfect" health as a means to control and punish ourselves, find our identity, and fill some big soul-holes.

- Option number two, we become so busy trying to self-medicate our wounds or disconnect from reality with things like work or romantic partners, that we completely neglect caring for our bodies.

- Or the final option, we use the act of eating food as our only solace from life's challenges.

Many of my clients will say they belong to this last group, they're self-proclaimed "emotional eaters." However, in my experience most are actually attempting to restrict and control their eating, and when this deprivation mindset naturally leads to an increased desire for "off-limit" foods and overeating, they wrongly label themselves emotional eaters.

Regardless, the root cause of all three of these scenarios is an unsatisfied heart, and the solution is the same. Stop seeking satisfaction in anything other than Christ; instead nourish your soul with the bread of life, and experience the lasting peace that comes with it. Christ alone has the power to break every stronghold.

EAT YOUR BREAD

Jesus said to them, "I am the bread of life; whoever comes to me shall not hunger, and whoever believes in me shall never thirst.

JOHN 6:35 ESV

Jesus likes to compare himself to food and drink—a lot. At first, it's a little weird. Full transparency here, even the disciples were put off by Him telling a crowd of His followers to, "eat His flesh and drink His blood." After a closer look, the food comparison starts to make sense. Only Jesus can satisfy our deepest cravings: cravings for love, righteousness, and purpose. Plus, coming from someone whose life's mission is to point people to God through the lens of nutrition, His words make for some pretty awesome teaching material.

When Jesus says anything over and over again, it's like He's shouting, "Listen up, this is important!" In the gospel of John alone, he refers to himself as food and drink at least 17 times. Specifically, He calls himself the "bread of life." In the Hebrew culture bread represented much more than a loaf of yummy ground up grains and yeast. Bread signified all food, but even more, it stood for provision, sustenance, and health. In Jesus, God promises to provide, sustain, and heal His people. When Jesus says in the Sermon on the Mount, that those who hunger and thirst for righteousness will be satisfied, He's referring to Himself as the bread that will satisfy our desire for righteousness (Matthew 5:6). Now, when we take communion we eat the "bread" of His body and drink the "wine" of His blood, and we remember how He's blessed us and that our righteousness is because of Him and Him alone.

It's no surprise then, that when Jesus was teaching the Jewish people how to pray in Matthew 6:11, He includes the words, "Give us today our daily bread," in His prayer. He was setting the standard that we DAILY need to be reminded of His finished work on the cross, a work that yields forgiveness, provision, sustenance, and healing in our lives. If He wanted us to just remember it on Sundays or on Easter, He would have said give us our weekly or yearly bread. But no, just as we daily need physical food to keep our bodies alive and nourished, we need Jesus's food every moment of every day to nourish our soul and satisfy our deepest yearnings.

THE TRANSFORMATIVE POWER OF GRACE

If we truly want well-being in all its glorious forms: physical, psychological, emotional, and relational, we need to allow the gospel to set us free in every way possible. Our metamorphosis from enslaved to freed men and women happens as a result of grace, and the transformative power of grace begins and ends with Jesus. In fact, we can just go ahead and replace the word grace with His name, because Jesus IS grace. He's the unmerited, undeserved, unearned forgiveness and favor of God sent down for us.

Yes, I do realize I'm being repetitive with this whole grace thing. But the reason I mention it over and over again is this: there is NOTHING like a deep revelation of God's grace—His unearned and unchanging love—to break the chains of religion and shake off every weight that hinders us. The reality is that God loves every human being with the same intensity, whether a broken-down drug addict or a lead pastor of a booming church, we are all His favorites. And even though you may be 20 years into your faith and winning souls to Jesus with your life, you are no better and no more loved by God than the husband and father caught in adultery. Hearing this truth for the first time wrecked me. If I'm being honest, I knew I wasn't perfect, but I certainly thought I was better than *that* person down the road who did *that* terrible thing.

When I first believed in Jesus, I thought I understood grace. But as time went on and I no longer struggled with some of the more "unsavory" sins (as if any sin is better than another) I started to think I'd earned God's blessings and favor whereas other people with "worse sin problems" did not. You see, I was still holding onto a deep seeded insecurity that God's love was earned through good deeds. And because I believed this for myself, I found it hard to extend grace to other people I didn't think deserved it.

Grace started and stopped at salvation for me. Yes, I was going to heaven, and I'd cleaned up some of my behaviors on the outside, but my heart still struggled with the same pride and insecurity. It wasn't until I started believing the whole truth of grace that my desires and perceptions began to transform. I realized God's standard is not good, it's perfection; even being a "good Christian" was like dirty rags to him. The only reason I, or anyone else, was or is blessed is because of His amazing grace, because of Jesus's perfect sacrifice, so that no one may boast. I now understand that I haven't earned a thing and never will, so I can no longer expect others to earn grace either. God doesn't want a shout out every now and then, and He certainly doesn't want my religious activities and self-improvement efforts. He wants to be the sole captain of my life. He wants to take me places only He can, so that Jesus gets all the glory.

Through His life and ministry, grace was the primary truth that Jesus taught. He came and revealed just how impossible it is to measure up to God's perfect standard and how desperately we need a savior for justice to be satisfied–grace.

He lived the perfect human life through the power of the Holy Spirit in Him, the same spirit who gave Him instructions about God's will and empowered Him to perform miracles, miracles that He performed for sinners because of their faith, not their great character—grace.

Despite His complete innocence, He was killed as one who was guilty of the entire world's sins in order to pay the FULL price for our mistakes past, present, and future—grace.

On the third day God raised him from the dead as a picture of our new life and victory over death—grace.

And as a final act, after he ascended into heaven, Jesus sent the Holy Spirit to every believer, so that we too could have God living in us, instructing us, empowering us, and giving us the authority to heal the sick and overcome the world—grace.

This message of grace, which has been preached for 2,000 years is so transformative that it makes enemies of God and murderers of His people into martyrs and preachers of the truth. Saul of Tarsus was one such man. He hated Christians and zealously persecuted them. Until one day, Jesus revealed himself to Saul and taught him the truth. At that time, Saul was given a new name as a reflection of his new identity in Christ, Paul.

Paul went on to become the most prolific apostle in the early church, writing at least thirteen of the twenty-seven books of the New Testament. And what was Paul's primary message? We are made righteous by grace through faith, not by works; we are dead to the law and alive to Jesus! I can't help but think that Paul's fervor for the grace of God resulted from the fact that he understood just how badly he personally needed grace, maybe even more so than other disciples. After all, he was an enemy of the kingdom of God and grace, and a spiritual encounter with Jesus turned him into a prophet to the nations for all time. You want to talk about total transformation, Paul's your guy.

The truth of grace is the singular teaching that Jesus was referring to when He said in John 8:31-32, "If you hold to my teaching, you are really my disciples. Then you will know the truth, and the truth will set you free." If we hold onto the truth of grace, even when it goes against everything we've learned out in the world, and especially when we mess up, then we will experience ultimate freedom in Christ. On the contrary, if we treat grace like a one-time loan Christ made on our lives that has to be paid back, we will remain in bondage to our debt. Spending our lives trying to prove to the world, to God, and to ourselves that we really are saved, that we really do deserve grace is not God's idea of abundant life.

As far as health is concerned, believing the whole truth of grace means we understand that we do not have to strive and work for God's best. He wants to bless us with health. Let me say that again for the people in the back, God wants you to be healthy! God does not cause sickness or disease. He designed you to be healthy and whole. Health is a blessing that God freely gives to His children. We get in the way of His blessings, not by having poor self-control or eating the wrong foods, but by not understanding His grace. Our belief that rules and creation are somehow the answer to our problems drives us to strive after health and not God. I believe that God is calling us to slow down enough to seek Him and His will for our life. As we do this, we allow him to speak to us about all things, including our physical health.

He will guide you in every area, including what to eat, when to eat, and when to stop eating. He doesn't do it through a set of rules. Because let's be honest, we can't even follow rules we set for ourselves. In fact, setting rules like "I will not eat donuts this week" almost always guarantees we'll break them. God knows this about us and so He chooses to lead us by His spirit, day-by-day and moment-by-moment. Similarly, God doesn't reveal everything that's going to happen in our future or along the journey, because He knows we'd get in our own way. He calls us to trust Him instead, to trust that He will take care of us despite the imperfect world we live in.

If we are quiet enough to hear Him and confident in His finished work, we will be able to discern the truth He's telling us from the lies of the enemy. Our thoughts will no longer be consumed by food and body image, and because of this, our mind won't continue to get in the way of caring for our body and following its signals.

Eventually, He will change our habits to align with what's best for us. He will give us freedom from the fear of food, but before He can clean up the outside, He needs our hearts! 1 John 3 tells us that when we remember that God is much more merciful than our own condemning conscience, that he knows us and accepts us fully, then our hearts will no longer condemn us. When this happens, John tells us we will have a bold freedom to speak to God face-to-face and believe that whatever we ask for, we will receive. What a promise!

The key to obtaining this bold freedom is remembering God's grace, mercy, and love. Feeding off this truth, over and over again, is the essence of the empowered Christian life. It results in a quiet and confident soul, one that seeks the best for oneself and others, one that is open to hearing from the Spirit.

GO WHERE YOUR SOUL IS CALLED

Rooted in grace and confidence, we start to grow from the inside out into the person that God always intended for us to be. While all of us are being transformed into the image of Christ, each of us has a unique role, viewpoint, or characteristic we bring to the world. Part of soul nourishment is feeding our gifting with the food it needs to grow and bring God glory. For instance, if you feel uniquely called to write, let's say you enjoy it and God has given you some measure of talent in that area, then soul-care might mean starting a daily writing practice. Alternatively, if you have a passion for music, but you've never learned an instrument, soul-care might be taking guitar lessons. Maybe you aren't sure what God is calling you to, in that case soul-care may look like making more time to hear from him.

Frederick Beuchner defines calling in his book, *Wishful Thinking,* writing, "The place God calls you to is the place where your deep gladness and the world's deep hunger meet."[3] Your calling is not necessarily what you think you *should* be doing, but what you enjoy doing. God puts desires in our heart for a reason. Similarly, He directs our steps to nurture our talents, and He brings certain people into our lives to call out our gifting. Soul-care means trusting in him enough to take a step of faith into your calling. For many, this means cutting out the things that are inhibiting you from walking in your purpose. This might mean taking a pay cut to start a more fulfilling job or giving up a volunteer activity on the weekends to spend more time with your family. Some of the unnecessary activities that take up our time are good things, but if they aren't in God's plan for our life, they gotta go. If we're honest, a lot of these activities stem from our striving to make God's blessings happen on our own terms.

Remember Abraham, the guy in the Old testament who had a baby at 100 years old and birthed the nation of Israel? He and his wife, Sarah, received a promise from God for a child in their old age and they believed Him for it. But at a point in the twenty-five-year waiting process they decided God's timing wasn't working for them. In order to force the issue of a son, Sarah gave her maidservant, Hagar to her husband to sleep with. What a mess. Low and behold, Hagar conceived. The maidservant resented Sarah for what she'd done and Sarah resented her. By trying to make God's blessing happen, Sarah hurt people and created strife. When Sarah finally did have a baby, there was enmity between her son, Isaac, and the son of her maidservant, Ishmael, so she sent Hagar and the boy away into the wilderness.

Listen, what Sarah did was wrong. She failed to trust what God had said and instead tried to control the situation in a terrible way. But the story isn't about Sarah, it's about God's faithfulness to stay true to His promises and work everything for good, despite our human failings. God saw Hagar and her son and the injustice done to them and He provided for them; He blessed Ishmael with a nation of his own. He also remained true to His promise to Abraham and gave him a son through Sarah in their old age.

God works everything together for our good (Romans 8: 28), but how much hurt could we save ourselves, and others, if we just trusted His way and stopped trying to make everything happen on our own.

SELF-CARE REDEEMED

Nourishing your soul first means being aware of what you need, mentally, emotionally, and spiritually and responding accordingly. The opposite of this occurs when we suppress our thoughts, emotions, and needs until it's too late and we're having to do damage control. This is where the majority of us camp out, in this uncontrolled, reactive state where we let our thoughts and emotions go unchecked until they force themselves to the surface and cause a knee-jerk reaction. This reaction is often not the type of behavior we want to keep around. Let me give you an example. When my husband and I were newly married I had certain expectations of him. I believed the man should help with the dishes; it's what my dad did, so why would it be any different in my new home? Well, my husband didn't grow up the same way I did, so he wasn't too concerned with the cleaning up after dinner. Instead of telling him I needed help, I let my resentment build and build every time I'd see a dirty dish pile, until one night I unloaded on him. It was not pretty. If I had told him what I needed sooner, and how I felt, I could have prevented that type of reaction. It's the same with our caring for our souls, and ultimately our bodies. We need to be conscious of our thoughts and emotions so we can give them to the Lord and address them early on.

Unless you're living in a bubble, you've probably heard the term self-care and you might be thinking this whole soul-care thing sounds similar. It is. Only, I like to think of soul-care as the redeemed version of self-care. Often times self-care comes across as this thing you do just because someone told you to do it. We hear people talk about taking bubble baths, reading a book, and getting their nails done. And sure, maybe this is what you need, and there's certainly no shame in a good Mani Pedi! But if the self-care method you're employing doesn't address the root need of your soul, it's a temporary coping mechanism at best. Hear me, coping mechanisms aren't bad, they just aren't a permanent solution. Soul-care says, I need Jesus first and foremost to heal all my wounds and remind me of my place as His child. Next, it allows the Holy Spirit to speak and guide us towards what we really need and what we're called to do. In response, we can choose to take an intentional step towards healing and transformation and calling.

Think about it, if you had a broken leg that needed surgery wouldn't you rather have the surgery, heal your broken bones, and continue to walk towards your destination than refuse surgery and limp around with your broken leg in a cast forever? That's what happens when we nourish our soul with the One who heals, satisfies and encourages, as opposed to relying on spiritual band aids. So, rip off that band aid, bring your brokenness to him, and find refreshment for your soul—you're going to need it. We're about to dive into the truth about food, exercise, and body image in the following chapters and you're going to want to put on your new identity before you take this step forward.

REFLECTION QUESTIONS

1. Where has the health of your soul (mind, will, and emotions) been related to your physical health?

2. Do you know anyone with Godly contentment? What's different about them? How does the revelation of God's grace affect your view of yourself and your life?

3. What gifts and talents has God given you? What desires has he placed in your heart? Do you see where these might align into a calling? If not, pray and ask God to reveal where he's calling you.

4. What is God calling you to cut out of your life in order for you to care for your soul better? What is he calling you to start?

Chapter 3

CONDEMNATION'S ROLE IN HEALTH & WELLNESS

"There is therefore now no condemnation for those who are in Christ Jesus. For the law of the Spirit of life has set you free in Christ Jesus form the law of sin and death."

ROMANS 8: 1-2 NIV

SHAME & DEATH ENTERED TOGETHER

Have you ever wondered how or why there's so much sickness in the world, especially among believers? How do we continue to get sick and struggle with chronic disease when the majority of what Jesus did on earth was heal the sick?

I don't pretend to have all the answers to this, but I do know God is our healer. Even though we experience sickness on this side of eternity, He has promised to be our deliverer. I've heard people say that healing miracles only happened in the early church, with Jesus and His disciples, that healing is not for us today. But I refuse to believe that.

I have seen healing happen in an instant with prayer. Likewise, I have seen it happen over time with persistent faith, despite circumstances. The Bible very clearly says that by Jesus's stripes we ARE healed (Isaiah 53:5). Not we will be healed if we beg God for it or if we eat clean enough; simply, we are healed. So, either you believe those words or you don't, but I know they are true. The good news is that they are true for you too, as you stand on them and on the faithfulness of Jesus' finished work, His grace.

So much of our focus and idolatry of eating and exercise is rooted in our desire to be healthy, or rather fear of becoming unhealthy. On the outside, it seems justified. Read every other news headline and you'll find something about the latest dietary toxin or lifestyle caused disease. Right after the title of the article follows paragraphs full of scare tactics and the latest crazy cleanse or set of dietary rules to save yourself from that particular disease. Of course, these articles play on our fear, and we eat it up! And while taking care of our bodies is a good thing, there is no diet or exercise plan that can save us. Our savior has a name and His name is Jesus. And so, this chapter on shame and sickness starts with hope, based on a promise, that we, as believers, need to take hold of if we're ever going to see the full goodness of God on this side of eternity. This is the truth: God is our healer.

We can believe God is our healer and still steward the bodies He gave us, knowing that it is not our perfect actions that make us healthy, but Jesus' sacrifice and God's hand on us that gives us health. It is God's will that we would be healthy here on earth. He does not send sickness or disease, but He does deliver us from them. Similarly, the

Bible doesn't tell us to neglect our bodies, ignore our diagnoses and symptoms, and refuse medical care, but it does tell us that faith means we call things that are not as though they were (Romans 4:17). So, if we believe that we are healed because of the promise of God in Christ, we call ourselves healed even when we do not yet see the symptoms of complete healing. And we continue to obey and trust God in faith while we wait for Him. Practically, this means we continue to care for our bodies without worrying and stressing that what we eat or do with them is more important than God's healing power. This principle holds true in every area of our lives, in our finances, our marriages, and our relationships with our children. We pray and we believe for healing in these areas, because we believe in a God who heals.

Faith is the evidence of things hoped for, but not yet seen! I did not set out to write a book on healing, but I know that when you see God as one who heals, it's a lot easier to put food and exercise back in their rightful place and put God in His. If you are struggling with symptoms and diagnosis of disease, and healthy eating has become your main hope, I want to encourage you by reminding you that our Father is faithful to heal you completely. He is way better than any clean eating regimen. After all, He made food and our bodies—how can the creation be better than its creator?

Even still, our mind searches for a reason, an understanding of how sickness and pain entered the world and why we're so affected by it.

If you ask Google, you'll find a million different answers out there, but if you look at the Bible narrative, everything was perfect until Adam and Eve ate from the tree of the knowledge of good and evil. When they doubted God's goodness, believing the lie from the enemy that God was holding out on them, and acted out of this distrust, eating from the tree of the knowledge of good and evil, sin and death entered the world. For God had commanded them, "You may surely eat of every tree of the garden, but of the tree of the knowledge of good and evil you shall not eat, for in the day that you eat of it you shall surely die (Genesis 2:16-17 ESV)." Think about that. God said that in the day that they ate the fruit they would surely die, yet if we know the rest of the story, we know that Adam and Eve continued to live on the earth for many years afterwards. Why then does God say that they will die that day?

Let's look at the narrative.

When God found Adam and Eve they were ashamed of eating from the tree and awake to the fact that they were naked, so they hid. Adam and Eve were now painfully aware of right and wrong, good and evil. They were aware of their own failings and that their disobedience deserved punishment. With this knowledge, came something else—condemnation.

Merriam Webster defines the verb condemn as the act of declaring something to be "reprehensible, wrong, or evil usually after weighing evidence and without reservation; to pronounce guilty."[1] In other words, condemnation is a constant awareness of our own guilt; it's a death sentence hanging over our heads. Notice God did not have to condemn Adam and Eve, they did it themselves. They obtained the knowledge of good and evil by eating the fruit of the tree, and their eyes were opened to their wrong act.

They hid because they were afraid, afraid of the punishment they now knew they deserved.

What follows after God finds Adam and Eve hiding is the consequence for their actions, the curse. The woman is told that she will have pain in childbearing and that her desire shall be contrary to her husband, but that he shall rule over her. The man is told that he will work the ground in pain and eat of it in pain, that he shall eat by the sweat of his brow and return to dust at the end of his days. In other words, death and pain entered the world and our perfect health was disrupted.

But notice that before health was disrupted, their consciences were disrupted; they were seared with the knowledge of sin, they were ashamed. Peace was taken from them as a result of their disobedience and new awareness of good and evil. Condemnation, guilt, and shame entered the human experience, and death quickly followed.

No, Adam and Eve didn't drop dead on the day they ate of the tree, but if you know anything about the human body, you know that every day our bodies are dying. In that moment, their hearts began beating toward an end. As we age our genes divide and shorten, our body systems don't work as well as they once did, and our heart beats one beat closer to its physical limit. Of course, there are things we can do to slow down the dying process, as well as things we do to speed it up. Interestingly enough many of the lifestyle "remedies" we practice in order to live longer are aimed at doing one thing: reducing stress

STRESS, HEALTH, & THE GOSPEL

The results of Adam and Eve's sin was shame and toil, a downcast spirit and heavy labor. Today we lump these states of being under the category of stressful. And while condemnation might not be a familiar term, stress most certainly is. We have all kinds of stress in this world. We have physical stress from over exercising; lack of sleep; poor nutrition; injury; alcohol, tobacco, and drug use; lack of movement; and inadequate hydration. Then there is emotional and psychological stress brought on by worry, anxiety, overcommitting and overworking, broken relationships, fear, and shame. And the list goes on. You name it—we all experience stress this side of heaven.

Whether it's physical stress and inflammation or mental stress, we're obsessed with decreasing it, dealing with it, and studying it because we know it plays a central role in our physical health. We are becoming increasingly aware of the link between stressful living and the risk of disease.

At the root of all this stress—emotional, mental and physical—is shame, un-forgiveness, and condemnation. Our belief that we are guilty and have to earn love, forgiveness, right standing, and worth drives us to mental unrest (stress), to neglect and tune out from our bodies (stress), to overwork (stress), and to bitterness and relational divides (stress). And what's sad, is condemnation comes so easy to us. It's natural. Ever since the garden we've become pros at recognizing our guilt and shortcomings. And if we don't recognize it, the enemy loves to remind us.

The good news is we don't *have* to live with a guilty conscience. Jesus came to live the perfect life in total surrender to the Father's will. He fulfilled every iota of the law of good and evil. He gave complete control to the Father unto death, giving Himself over to be beaten, scourged, and crucified on the cross as the punishment for every single sin, past, present, and future.

If you've been around the church any, this may sound pretty basic. But this is still the most powerful truth of all time. If we really believed that we were forgiven all of our sins, if we believed that Christ paid it all and God's blessings are now ours in Christ, we would be changed. The knowledge of this would give us peace, a clear conscience, and a thankful heart. It would set us free from striving and drive us to surrender all to our loving father. Yet, we hold on to shame. We forgive others, but we rarely forgive ourselves. Shame and striving are second nature to us.

Not too long ago, I was on a walk with my friend and our three children, all under the age of five. In typical fashion, the kiddos started getting restless, especially Leena, the four-year old. The sweet girl started begging her mama to let her push the double stroller with her eighteen-month-old brother in tow. Despite her mom telling her no, Leena insisted, declaring, "I got it," pushing the stroller out from under her mama. Not two steps in, the entire stroller, baby brother and all, toppled over onto the cement sidewalk.

Isn't that just so typical of human behavior? God says, "Not yet sweetie," knowing that there are things we must learn, and growing that has to happen, before we can have what we're asking for. But we proudly talk back, "Don't worry Father, I got this, I'll do it on my own. I'll help you out." But we never really get too far on our own, do we? Or maybe we do, but it ends in disaster. Like a little child, we see our error and we suddenly feel pretty silly, or worse, we feel utterly ashamed and afraid, afraid of the punishment we believe we deserve.

After the stroller hit the ground, things happened pretty quickly, Tarren, my friend, stooped down and grabbed her little boy, who despite being shaken up, was injury free. Next, she righted the stroller and looked for Leena. Leena was five feet away, hiding behind the only tree on the path. She was visibly ashamed, upset, and fearful of getting in trouble. Tarren spoke to her calmly, assuring Leena that her brother was okay. In the most non-accusatory voice, Tarren said, "We need to stay in the stroller and let mommy push it until we get to the car, okay?" I remember being impressed by her calm and gracious response, and a little guilty, thinking about how I likely wouldn't have responded so well. But despite all this, Leena was ashamed.

Hiding and crying turned to defensive insults as she told her mom, very matter-of-factly, "Daddy is my favorite daddy." Try not to smile at that. After this, her mom walked over, bent down, and gently talked to her until she was willing to get back in the stroller. All was well. No punishment, just love and understanding.

Our automatic response to messing up is to feel shame and fear, fear of the punishment we believe we deserve—in other words, condemnation. Just like Leena, we hide from our heavenly father, afraid that He'll punish us severely for our disobedience. We might even start blaming Him for our mistake, irrationally throwing out insults and excuses. But His response is always the same. With grace and compassion, He picks us back up and takes us back to where we belong.

God calls us His children and reminds us He has already sent Jesus to die on the cross as the punishment for all of our sins, past, present, and future. He reminds us that He no longer remembers our sins, nor holds them against us, but that He loves us and simply wants what's best for us. His love is perfect, and there is no fear in perfect love, because fear suggests punishment. But God's love says that there is no longer any condemnation (no guilty sentence and resultant punishment) for those who are in Christ Jesus. Further, there is no more curse, because Jesus redeemed us from the curse by becoming a curse for us (Galatians 3:13).

After Adam and Eve sinned and the curse entered the world, being the merciful, loving father that He is, God made the very first sin offering of animals for their atonement. He clothed Adam and Eve with the skins, covering their nakedness and making a way for them to continue in relationship with Him. This was a shadow of the ultimate sacrifice that was to come.

God did one more thing: He kicked Adam and Eve out of the garden of Eden—another mercy—lest they eat of the tree of life and live forever in their current sin conscious state.

God already knew that one day He'd send the perfect sin offering. He'd send his son, Jesus, to give us eternal, permanent forgiveness. This forgiveness, when we believe it for ourselves, gives us a clear conscience. A conscience that allows us to sit at God's feet in peace, full of trust, full of expectation, like a child, ready to learn and receive all the good things a loving parent can give.

Health is one of those good things, one of the many gifts God longs to provide for us if we would just let Him, if we would just accept His grace on our lives and stop trying to earn His blessings through works. That type of striving only results in burnout and stress out.

The truth of the gospel sets us free to rest in God's love for us, and in rest we find peace and healing. If all we ever do is meditate on this truth, we will never become tired of it. It is the foundation for everything else, including how we nourish our bodies.

It's my prayer that this message sink in like never before and you will be transformed from the inside out. And then eating, food, exercise, all these things, will come easily, almost accidentally. So, it is with a grace conscience and an open heart, that we move forward into deeper and deeper freedom in Christ!

REFLECTION QUESTIONS:

1. What past mistakes or current sins play over and over in your mind? Is there anything you believe you've done that God doesn't forgive or that he's somehow punishing you for? That's not the God of the gospel. Every time your mind goes to the place of shame, I challenge you to confess: I am forgiven in Jesus name and thank God for this forgiveness.

2. How has your own shame or guilt caused you stress? What would it feel like to not worry about your shortcomings?

3. How do you offer forgiveness to other people? How do you offer forgiveness to yourself? Are they different? Can you say, "I forgive you" out loud, to yourself?

4. How has striving to receive God's blessing, love, or worth affected your life? What can you let go of and trust God with when you truly believe He sees you as forgiven?

Chapter 4

OWNING YOUR TRUE IDENTITY & WORTH

"Therefore, if anyone is in Christ, the new creation has come:[1] The old has gone, the new is here!"

2 CORINTHIANS 5:17 NIV

Have you ever had someone look you in the eye and calmly ask, "Who are you?" as if the question was so simple. I remember the first time someone asked me that question: I was in college. Initially, my mind went blank as I grappled for an answer. I was scrambling, racking my brain for words to sum up my identity. Eventually, I did respond. I recited a list of my accomplishments and group memberships in order of perceived importance, the way I imagine a neatly organized resume would read.

But those things weren't my identity; they were just activities I did and people I associated with. At the time though, they were the things that gave me value. Like any foundation formed outside of Christ, mine eventually crumbled, piece by piece. First it was my swimming career that ended, I was no longer Aubrey, Swim Team Captain, Athlete Extraordinaire. Next, student life was stripped from me; I could no longer use my classroom performance to define my identity or measure my worth. Then it was the job I wanted that was taken, and what was left was just my obsession with food and exercise. But life got in the way of that too, or rather I like to think God did. It was impossible to eat "perfectly" and exercise daily with real life demands: work, marriage, and a tiny budget. What was left was just a broken-down girl with, seemingly, no identity or worth. But how many of us know that God uses our most broken moments to teach us about His grace and our place as His children?

Piece by piece, as I surrendered to my only remaining hope—Jesus, He picked me up and taught me about His love and His purpose for my life. He taught me that the things I found my value in were garbage compared to what He offers. I look back at that girl and I'm saddened. I wish, so desperately, that from the beginning I would have set my worth on Jesus's love for me. But for some of us stubborn folk, it takes all our false hopes being dashed to see the one true hope. As long as we continue to turn to something other than God to give us meaning and value, as often as we try to do everything on our own without His help, He lets us. God values freedom, so He allows us to choose our own way, even if it's the wrong choice, all while pursuing us anyway.

Your heavenly Father is calling to you now, even in the midst of your pursuit for happiness outside of Him. He's showing you His great love and the brokenness of the thing or system you're seeking value from. But He does not control our choices, He gives us free will. We can use it to surrender to Him or we can choose to keep on keepin' on with our to-do lists, diet plans, controlling attitudes, and pursuing approval from other people. I can promise you this, when you give all that up, when you choose to surrender all the outcomes of your life to Him, His burden is easy, far easier than the self-help program you're following and far easier than carrying the world on your shoulders. What's more, His outcomes are good; every time His plan for us is better than what we could ever imagine for ourselves.

A NEW CREATION BY GRACE THROUGH FAITH

Hear me out, surrendering to Jesus does not mean begrudgingly performing religious activities because you know it's the right thing to do and hoping that God will reward you for your model citizenship. That is religion, or legalism, and what Jesus spent the majority of His time on earth chastising the Pharisees for. Surrendering to Jesus means believing and confessing that you are made new, righteous, and holy by His blood and sacrifice. It's laying aside your old identity—the one that was ruled by shame and self-obsession—and putting on your new identity, one that is motivated by God's love for you and empowered by His Holy Spirit in you. You are not saved by unmerited grace, only to try earning God's favor through good behavior. You are a new creation the moment you believe and confess with your mouth that Jesus is Lord, and you continue to be a new creation every day from that moment forward. The only work you have to do is to continue to believe this truth despite what the world looks like or the circumstances around you. This is the daily work of a believer, it's what Paul is referring to when he implores Christians to "fight the good fight of faith" in 1 Timothy 6:12.

The beauty of believing this truth is that you will begin to act like it. To many rule followers grace is scary. I find people asking, "Won't we just keep on sinning if grace means we are righteous no matter what we do?" or "How will we find the motivation to not act badly if we aren't focusing on the Ten Commandments or constantly examining our behaviors and motives?" This is religion's favorite argument, but the reality is so much better. When we are set free from constantly looking at our own sin, and instead focus on Jesus and who He says we are, we start to feel loved, and we begin to seek him and listen to his Holy Spirit for guidance. As we yield moment-by-moment to the Spirit's work in us, we begin to change from the inside out. We do things because God asks us to do them, not because we're trying to prove ourselves, earn righteousness, or make up for our sin. Outward change comes with simple obedience to the Spirit's leading, with barely any conscience effort of our own.

Have you ever met someone who has been truly transformed by the grace of God? The biggest transformation stories don't come from people who were simply trying to get their act together, they come from people who knew they couldn't do it on their own, who recognized without a shadow of a doubt that they were sinners, that what they were doing wasn't working, who were desperate to get out from under the weight of their current identity, desperate to have someone really know them and love them anyways. The moment someone shares with that person they have worth and value beyond measure, that they are completely new in Christ, that they don't have to earn a thing—that's when powerful transformation takes place. It's not when someone comes and points out their sin that they see Jesus, no, that only serves to deepen shame and hopelessness. We are saved by God's grace through faith in Christ, and not by works, so that no man may boast.

I have been a professing Christian for as long as I can remember. At the age of 4 I knelt beside my mom and asked Jesus to come into my heart. I grew up in church. My parents attended a Christian university where they met, and my dad was even an evangelical pastor for several years. I knew to love Jesus because he'd forgiven my sins, and I certainly tried my best. I'd heard all the Bible stories and I knew all the commandments. Slowly but surely, Jesus PLUS rule following became my primary belief system. As a child, I began focusing on doing good, obeying the rules so that I could please my parents and God, so things would go well for me. For the most part, this belief system served me well, sheltered by my parents and full of childlike innocence—until of course, it didn't.

I grew up, I made mistakes, both big and small. And because of my vast "church wisdom" of right and wrong, sin and the commandments, I felt ashamed. I resolved to "do better," but eventually I'd slip back into the same mistakes. Eventually I just let those mistakes rule me, I made concession for my sin. It was impossible to get better after all—this was me. The enemy whispered that over and over. For a long while, this is how I lived. At times, I'd hear an inspiring sermon or get hooked up with a good group of friends and make decisions to get out of certain sins. I'd "clean up" my act. But the root of my beliefs was still a false theology, one where I worked and God nodded his head from afar, yay or nay.

There were two significant seasons in my life that ultimately shaped my faith and transformed me into the person I am today: a woman freed and on mission. And no, neither of those seasons involved getting an accountability partner to point out my obvious breaking of the commandments or ask me how I'd sinned. The second season of transformation happened after I was married and birthed a vision for this book. But the first occurred earlier (as firsts normally do), right after I'd deeply hurt the person I loved most, my soon to be fiancé, and now husband.

I am not proud of who I was in college, and I don't write this to glorify or even justify my selfish actions at the time, but rather to demonstrate how broken I was and how good God is.

During the early years of us dating neither my husband or me were solidly planted and convinced of God's grace. I didn't think of myself as loved, accepted, or living for purpose. Rather I thought of myself like an athlete who was constantly trying out for the team, continually vying for position with God and with people.

If you've ever sought fulfillment in your performance or in your ability to please people then you know it never ends well. The praises from others and accolades are never enough. Before you know it you're sacrificing your relationships, your peace, and your own soul in pursuit of the next thing that will satisfy. That was me. I found myself chasing down the attention of other guys in the midst of dating my husband. It was all fine and harmless until one day it went too far and I crossed a line. The saddest part was I loved my boyfriend. I knew I wanted to marry him, but deep down I had cracks, false beliefs about God and myself that "finding the one" could never fix.

I'll never forget the shame I felt sitting on the floor the next day in my bathroom, in disbelief at the person I'd become and the things I was capable of doing, supposedly a Christian and yet, still so self-centered and powerless to my sin. I kept thinking there was no way he'd forgive me for this, no way he'd still want to be with me after I'd hurt him so badly. I remember crying out honestly for the first time in a long time, "Father help me, I am sorry, I don't know why I do these things but I need you. I need Jesus."

As painful as those next few days were, admitting my sin and asking for forgiveness from the love of my life, they were the turning point for everything. Rather, the grace I was offered by one person was the turning point for everything. Although I'd hurt him badly, my amazing, wonderful man showed me so much love and forgiveness. That kind of radical, undeserved mercy and grace hits you hard. It pointed me to the mercy and grace God gives us through Jesus. It pointed me to the gospel I'd heard as a child but had somehow failed to remember up until that point in my life.

I began to feel thankful that I could not be good or please God, or anyone, by my own self-effort. For the first time ever, I knew deep down I couldn't live life, and live it well, on my own, and that I needed God's grace. I started to see myself in a new light—in the light of Jesus' sacrifice. I began to trust God and seek Him and His truth more; I began to be transformed.

Seven years later our story looks so different than the broken girl on the bathroom floor could have imagined. As I write this, Dwayne and I have been married six wonderful years. We have one beautiful son whose very name, Judah, means praise God, and we're expecting a second child. A day doesn't pass where I'm not thankful for Dwayne and our marriage, which is one of the greatest blessings of my life. God took my brokenness and brought beautiful redemption out of it. His grace literally transformed me from the inside out.

Why is it so important for you to understand this in a book about eating? Because how we eat and care for our bodies—the amount of control we seek to have over them is directly tied to our belief about ourselves and about God. And Christians should have the best belief about themselves, not because we earned it or are better, but because the Bible says we are hidden in Christ, meaning our identity is wrapped up in His. Have you ever had someone mistake you for a friend or a family member? Sometimes it's flattering (and sometimes not so much). The beautiful thing about our identity being hidden in Christ is that God lumps us in with his son. How awesome is that? There is no one I'd rather be mistaken for than Jesus himself.

On the other hand, if you believe that your value is dependent on your good behavior or your performance, then you will not be able to take hold of the freedom found in knowing Jesus. However, if you believe that what God says about you is true, every day, all day, no matter what mistakes you may have made, that's where freedom lies. Freedom from anxiety, depression, low self-worth, and comparison; freedom from seeking acceptance from people; and freedom from food and body image bondage!

If you have the courage to believe what the Bible says about you, then you have an answer to the question, "Who are you?" The answer is this: you are a child of God, fearfully and wonderfully made, holy and set apart for a good purpose, called, made new, forgiven, a new creation, the righteousness of God, the light of the world.

You are a royal priesthood, favored, a friend of Jesus. In Him you are a conqueror, overcomer, the head and not the tail. By His stripes you are healed. You are a vessel of the Holy Spirit who gives you power, wisdom, and love, who reveals to you the truth in all things. In Christ, you are chosen, valuable, and dearly loved. But don't just take my word for it, look at these truths from scripture.

IDENTITY TRUTHS

- "You have all become true children of God by the faith of Jesus the Anointed One!" Galatians 3:26 TPT

- "I praise you, for I am fearfully and wonderfully made. Wonderful are your works; my soul knows it very well." Psalm 139:14 ESV

- "But you are a chosen race, a royal priesthood, a holy nation, a people for his own possession, that you may proclaim the excellencies of him who called you out of darkness into his marvelous light." 1 Peter 2:9 ESV

- "...and to put on the new self, created after the likeness of God in true righteousness and holiness." Ephesians 4:24 ESV

- "I, even I, am He who blots out your transgressions for My own sake; and I will not remember your sins." Isaiah 43:25 NIV

- "Therefore, if anyone is in Christ, the new creation has come: The old has gone, the new is here!" 2 Corinthians 5:17 NIV

- "No longer do I call you servants, for the servant does not know what his master is doing; but I have called you friends, for all that I have heard from my Father I have made known to you." John 15:15 ESV

- "These things I have spoken to you, so that in Me you may have peace. In the world you have tribulation but take courage; I have overcome the world." John 16:33 ESV

- "No, in all these things we are more than conquerors through him who loved us. For I am sure that neither death nor life, nor angels nor rulers, nor things present nor things to come, nor powers, nor height nor depth, nor anything else in all creation, will be able to separate us from the love of God in Christ Jesus our Lord." Romans 8:37-39 ESV

- "Therefore, as God's chosen people, holy and dearly loved, clothe yourselves with compassion, kindness, humility, gentleness and patience." Colossians 3:12 NIV

- "and with his wounds we are healed." Isaiah 53:5b ESV

- "For God will never give you the spirit of fear, but the Holy Spirit who give you mighty power, love, and self-control* [Revelation-light or instruction Aramaic]" 2 Timothy 1:7 TPT

As you embark on this journey to experience food and body image freedom, I encourage you to continually remind yourself of who you are in Christ. This might mean you have a daily practice of repeating scripture affirmations in front of the mirror. It could look like taping reminders on your wall or making a background image for your phone, whatever it is, keep the Word front and center, listening to and believing the truth of your identity in Christ.

The world wants to dissuade you of your value, to continually point you to your flaws and offer false solutions. In knowing who you are, and who it is you trust in, you begin to think and act from a place of already being enough. No longer needing to earn anything, you'll start to notice new desire and new energy to live out who God designed you to be. You'll notice a sense of peace, and a desire to take care of your body in a balanced and enjoyable way, so that you can live life fully. I think we call this being grounded, content, confident, and empowered. How does that sound for a life resume?

REFLECTION QUESTIONS:

1. What activities, relationships, or things are you finding your identity & worth in other than Christ? Think about the things you rely on to make you feel happy or "in control" during a tough time.

2. What scriptures/identifiers in Christ speak to your heart?

3. How can you remind yourself daily of your great worth to God?

4. How does knowing your identity change your view of your health and your body?

Chapter 5

LAYING ASIDE THE PURSUIT OF WEIGHT LOSS

"Come to me, all you who labor and are heavy burdened, and I will give you rest."

MATTHEW 11:28 ESV

Heavy. I felt heavy. Heavy with the undue weight of shame and disgust I felt about my body changing, heavy under the self-induced pressure to look a certain way and weigh a certain number. So, I did the thing, I stepped on the bathroom scale. Immediately, I cringed at the number I saw. It was the most I'd weighed in my entire adult life. I could feel the disappointment and anxiety coming on, like a wave of tension crashing over my body. Ironically enough, I had been taking good care of myself, resting, eating all food groups regularly, drinking water, and taking prenatal vitamins; it's what you're supposed to do when you're trying to get pregnant. And it was working. I finally had a regular period for the first time in 5 years, making the chances of pregnancy pretty good.

But all of the sudden, the things I'd been doing to take care of my body appeared all wrong. I was "lazy, a glutton, self-indulgent, and stupid, and I needed to get back in line." I started planning the ways to make my diet "cleaner," deciding what food groups to cut, swearing off carbs and restaurants. Next, I started wracking my brain for ways to get more running in. The trouble was, we were busy. I was working 10-12 hour days at a place an hour away from our home. Going on an hour long run, my definition of exercise at the time, just wasn't going to happen for me. At this point, I became totally dejected. My mind spiraled into hopelessness. I would never look good, I would always struggle with eating and exercise, and it was all my husband's fault. If only he'd picked a different career, I wouldn't have to work so long, he wouldn't still be a student, and I would have time to work out. No, it was my fault, if only I had more self-control and more organizational, homemaker skills then we'd have home-cooked meals every night.

Wow. One arbitrary number on a little electronic device had so much power. Instead of glorying in the miracle that I could now conceive a child (something I had always wanted), I was degrading myself, and those closest to me. I actually began to plot the ways in which I could undo the healthy shift in my lifestyle that had produced a normal period in the first place (eating adequately, resting, decreasing exercise, etc.).

WHAT ARE YOU SEEKING?

My story is no different than countless others'. I see it on a daily basis with clients. Clients who are old, young, skinny, and fat, each have been obsessed with a number. Mostly it's a number on the scale, but sometimes it's their body fat percentage, calories for the day, pant size, social media followers, or macronutrient distribution. The number rules their decision to take care of their body or punish it, to meet their needs or to restrict, to speak positively to themselves or harshly.

If we aren't careful, I fear we'll never be able to consistently make nourishing choices for our bodies. If our focus is tied up in a number, we'll be discouraged by every normal fluctuation. Further, we'll be tempted to completely give up on ourselves when we find we can't control that number. So where is your focus? What are you are seeking?

If the answer is weight loss or health, there's most likely a deeper desire at play. For many of my clients, they're looking for acceptance, relationships, love, and approval. Others are seeking energy, long life, freedom from disease, and the ability to physically serve their families and God well.

Sometimes realizing where our focus lies is difficult. We may think we're focusing on Jesus, family, and health, but the enemy's deceptions are subtle. If in your mind, weight loss, or any other thing, has the ability to steal your joy or give you worth, then it's got your focus.

If you aren't sure what you're after, try this exercise. Write down several If/then statements on a piece of paper and follow them to their conclusion. For example, someone's if/then chain might read:

If I lose 20 lbs, then I'll be attractive.

If I'm attractive, then I'll get a spouse.

If I get a spouse, then I'll be content.

Your if /then may be totally different but look at where your if/then chain concluded. What are you really seeking? In the above example it's contentment, but how many of you know that's too tall of an order for a spouse to fill? It has to be God. Another common if/ then statement chain goes like this:

> If I eat only these certain foods and exercise this way, then
> I'll lose X number of pounds.

> If I lose X number of pounds, then I'll be skinny.

> If I'm skinny, then people will think I'm healthy.

> If they think I'm healthy, then they'll
> accept me, and I'll be normal.

We have to be able to lay down our concerns and desires at the feet of Jesus, and leave them there, this includes weight loss. We know that He desires to give you every good gift, which certainly includes health, but what if health has a whole lot less to do with our body size then we think?

WEIGHT LOSS DOESN'T EQUAL HEALTH

The problem with focusing on weight loss for health is that weight loss and health aren't synonymous. Popular culture tells us that a higher weight equals disease and a lower weight equals health, but this is a huge misrepresentation of the research. Let's look at Body Mass Index (BMI) for example. BMI is the ratio of a person's weight in kilograms to their height in meters squared. It was developed in the 19th century by a mathematician named Adolphe Quetelet, whose primary goal was to categorize the "average man." Later, it was adopted by a famed, and somewhat controversial nutrition researcher, Ancel Keys, to categorize different body sizes [1].

Eventually, researchers determined that higher BMIs (larger body weight in comparison to height), as well as lower BMIs (smaller body weight in comparison to height), were both risk factors for a number of diseases. Knowing that smaller and larger BMIs were risk factors for certain diseases helped researchers know what populations to screen.

For example, since lower BMIs are risk factors for malnutrition, the presence of these are a heads up for physicians to do further investigation and testing. Some of those who undergo testing have significant nutrient deficiencies and some do not. Therefore, a lower BMI is not equal to malnutrition. Malnutrition is equal to malnutrition. Similarly, a higher BMI is a risk factor for heart disease and diabetes. But not everyone with a higher BMI has heart disease or diabetes, not even close. In fact, there are many with a BMI of 30 or greater (what we define as obese) that are completely healthy. Meaning, they have no high blood pressure, no diabetes, or heart disease. This group has gotten so much attention recently, that we've come up with a term for them in the research, "metabolically healthy obese.[2]"

The American Medical Association has jumped the gun, in my opinion, classifying BMIs of 30 or greater as obesity and calling obesity a disease. As demonstrated above, just because you have a certain BMI does not mean you have a disease, or even that you're unhealthy. The presence of disease means you have a disease. The result of this leap in logic is that we're putting more and more value on weight, and less and less value on living a healthy lifestyle. This hasn't done a thing to decrease rates of chronic disease. In fact, rates of heart disease, diabetes, and the like have been steadily increasing, despite all-out efforts by researchers to develop and identify surgeries, diet pills, and eating regimens that produce long term weight loss.[3]

It's not to say that the desire to lose weight is wrong, but focusing on it has yet to be helpful. The reality is that almost all intentional weight loss efforts fail long term, with the overwhelming majority of those who lose weight gaining it back within three to five years, and up to two-thirds of dieters gaining even more weight than they lost. [4] Besides that, the majority of studies that see improvements in health markers (blood pressure, blood sugar, blood cholesterol, etc.) with short term weight loss don't control for the fact that study participants were often engaging in healthy behaviors like eating more fruits and vegetables, moving their bodies more, and drinking water.[4] In other words, weight loss gets all the credit for improving health when it's likely a result of lifestyle changes that would improve health, regardless of weight loss.

For instance, we know that when people increase healthy behaviors like adding more movement, eating fruits and vegetables, reducing alcohol intake, and stopping smoking, their rate of all-cause mortality decreases, even if their weight stays the same—even if their BMI says they're obese.5 If this is the case, then maybe, just maybe, weight loss isn't the panacea that our culture makes it out to be.

Isn't it just so typical, we've become so focused on what we believe is THE answer outside of Christ, THE means to all of our healing and happiness that even when it doesn't work, and all logic says stop this madness, we refuse to give in. We just stay at our post, stubbornly preaching the praises of weight loss, blaming the lack of results on the person and their poor discipline, instead of on the obviously flawed system. We humans have been pulling these shenanigans forever. Jesus actually addressed it with the lame man at the pool of Bethesda. You can read the whole story in John 5: 1–24.

Jesus visits the pool of Bethesda, which was known to have healing properties. He sees a crippled man lying by the pool, along with a multitude of others. Jesus knows the man has been lying there for thirty-eight years waiting for his chance to get in the water and be healed, yet He asks him this question, "Do you truly want to be healed?"

You just gotta love Jesus, He's not afraid to be blunt. He asks us straight up; do you want to be healed? Do you really want to give up this whole bondage to food and your body thing? Do you want to feel better, whole, unhindered? Look at the response Jesus receives at the pool.

"Sir, I have no way to get healed. I have no one to lower me into the water when the angel comes. As soon as I try to crawl to the edge of the pool, someone jumps in ahead of me." The man evades the question, instead giving the reason why he believes *can't* be healed. He is so focused on the means of his healing, or what he believes is the only way to be healed, that he can't see the truth—the healer is Jesus and He's standing right in front of him.

Many of us are crying out to God for health, confidence, affirmation, attention, and love. Maybe we're just crying out for weight loss. But God wants to know, do you really want to be healed? Do you really want recovery? We avoid him, complaining about all the reasons we can't eat clean enough, exercise long enough, or sleep deep enough. But He's not asking you if YOU can heal yourself on your own. He's asking if you want to be healed. If you do, then stop looking to the opinions of the world. Stop looking at what you lack, at your own shortcomings. Stop looking to clean eating and diets and weight loss. These are broken, fallen systems.

Look to the one who can do all things, who can overcome all things. Look to Jesus. Just like He told the crippled man to rise, take up his mat and walk, and he was healed, no healing pool necessary, He's telling you to throw off that old pursuit of weight loss, get rid of that next diet plan. Instead rise, walk, and know that He's got you. He is the one who redeems you and you need only pursue Him. Everything else will be added to you.

"So then, forsake your worries! Why would you say, 'What will we eat?' Or 'What will we drink?' Or 'What will we wear?' For that is what the unbelievers chase after. Doesn't your heavenly Father already know the things your bodies require? So above all, constantly chase after the realm of God's kingdom and the righteousness that proceeds from him. Then all these less important things will be given to you abundantly.

Refuse to worry about tomorrow, but deal with each challenge that comes your way, one day at a time."
Matthew 6:31-34 TPT

REFLECTION QUESTIONS:

1. How has your focus on your body, a number, or weight loss served you? How has it harmed you? What has it stolen from your life?

2. What are you waiting to do or become until you look a certain way/weigh a certain number? How can you take steps to do those things now?

3. What are you really hoping to accomplish with food/exercise/dieting, etc. Reference your if/then to specifically identify what your actions say you want to accomplish.

4. What would it look like for you to completely lay aside the pursuit of weight loss or a certain way of eating and exercising, and instead pursue Jesus?

Chapter 6

OF SPIRIT, SOUL, BODY & FLESH

"Stop imitating the ideals and opinions of the culture around you but be inwardly transformed by the Holy Spirit through a total reformation of how you think. This will empower you to discern God's will as you live a beautiful life, satisfying and perfect in his eyes."

ROMANS 12:2 TPT

A TRANSFORMATION STORY

Lily was a client of mine. She came to me by complete happenstance, looking for something or someone who would tell her the "right" way to eat, so she could finally lose weight and ultimately feel good about herself. Until that first phone call, she had no idea what a non-diet dietitian was, she just knew she needed professional help this time around and Google delivered my name to her search query.

The first bit of the phone call was the tricky part, but I was determined to share with her the entire truth of my philosophy before she committed to working with me. I explained that I didn't work with clients for the sole goal of weight loss, detailing my position that the pursuit of weight loss is rooted in restriction, dieting, and shame, and that it doesn't work. Her hesitation was palpable

I pressed on, explaining that I worked with people who were sick of dieting and ready to be free of the constant obsession, confusion, and guilt around food and exercise. Even over the phone I could tell this resonated with her deeply.

Lily ended up scheduling that first appointment and then another and another. We slowly worked to tear down the lies of diet culture that permeated every area of her life. She started to believe the truth that she was made for more than weight loss and that she could trust her body. Visibly, her demeanor began to change in sessions. She started dressing up, doing her makeup, and sitting taller. She was smiling and opening up, proclaiming the new freedom and energy she felt having let go of dieting. She was transforming.

It was in one of these sessions that Lily confided in me what she termed a "silly" secret fantasy of hers. She had imagined herself showing up to a dinner party, or an event, after not seeing her friends for a while. As she walked in, her friends congratulated her on her physical transformation, "Wow, you look amazing! What have you been doing? You're such an inspiration." The women were jealous of her and the men were envious of her husband. All in all, her fantasy was not unlike many contestants on popular weight loss shows.

In the social media generation, this fantasy would look like us posting a shocking before and after photo on

Instagram with the hashtag #transformationtuesday. Ideally, we'd receive praise and approval from all of our friends, followed by the accrual of new friends, new romantic pursuers, you name it.

Lily was not the first or the last client of mine to share a similar fantasy. The beauty of her story is that she was able to recognize the more important, permanent transformation that was taking place in her heart and mind and making its way into her body by means of improved health and energy.

As believers, we don't have to look forward to posting a #transformationtuesday picture on social media, we are continually being transformed.

What if we believed this? Would we live differently, pursue different things, and think better about ourselves?

The Bible tells us that when we believe in Jesus as our redeemer we are instantly made new. This transformation is a result of the Holy Spirit coming to live inside us the moment we believe. Let me take this opportunity to remind you that the Holy Spirit is for everyone; He lives inside everybody who professes Jesus as their savior. First, we are made righteous by grace through faith in Jesus and then Jesus sends the helper, the Spirit of truth, to teach us all things and guide us throughout life (John 14:16).

Yet, on the day you believe and receive the Holy Spirit, you will likely look and feel utterly the same; you might even continue acting the same. But the power is in the knowing and believing the truth. And over time, as our knowledge of Christ grows through the Holy Spirit's teaching, our inward transformation spreads to our entire being, as we yield to God's work within us. While much of this transformation is a complete mystery, I believe we can learn a great deal by looking deeper into the meanings of the words spirit, soul, body, and flesh.

THE MANY PARTS OF YOU

You've likely heard it said, "You are a spirit, you have a soul, and you live in a body," but what does that mean?

Let's start from the beginning of you, conception. From the time you were created in your mother's womb, your physical form was taking shape. This is your body and it encompasses the material aspects of you: skin, blood, bones, hair, muscles, organs, etc. This part of us is pretty well defined and the definition agreed upon. Our bodies are artfully designed by the creator to maintain and incline towards a state of health. Every physical instinct—to eat, to pee, to reproduce, to sleep—these were all given to us by a loving father in order to keep us alive, to give us pleasure, and to help us thrive.

You are not just your seen, physical body. There are intangible parts of you; you have a soul. This is where the definitions get tricky, but from my study of scripture and knowledge of psychology, I've formed an educated opinion on what I believe the soul is and what it does.

The soul houses our will, intellect, and emotions. It's where we hold our thoughts, ingrained responses, and unique personality tendencies. Our soul is shaped by our parents, genetics, our lived experiences, the environment around us, and the people we encounter. And as we discussed earlier, our thoughts (our soul) is intricately tied to our actions and connected to our physical well-being.

Existing within our soul is our conscience. This is the part of us that points out right from wrong, that tells us to act or not to act. The funny thing is, what your conscience tells you isn't always from God. Your conscience is susceptible to what you allow in and what you believe. For example, we may read a book about veganism and become convinced of its "rightness." Our conscience then downloads this information and dutifully convicts us of wrong when we eat contrary to this new set of guidelines. The result is often increased guilt and condemnation if we eat animal foods. But when we align this to God's word, which says all foods created by God are good, we often find that our food focused conscience is no longer based on God's word, but on man's opinions and personal convictions.

Hear me here, I'm not saying that everyone who follows a vegan diet is wrong or going against God's will. What God leads one person to do is between God and that person. And even if God doesn't lead the charge, we're free to follow our culturally informed, self-imposed convictions, but as we'll discuss later in the book, there is a way to listen to our body and the Spirit's leading with food that supplies much more freedom and grace than following the world's opinions and strict standards on eating.

Further, if freedom is our goal, then it's imperative that we align our thoughts, beliefs, and will (our soul) to the knowledge of Christ. In Romans 12:2 Paul urges us to stop imitating the outward world, with its rules and opinions. Instead, we must be inwardly transformed by the Holy Spirit through a total transformation of how we think (our soul). This brings us to the deepest part of you, the essence of who you are eternally, your spirit.

The spirit is probably the most difficult component to talk about because it runs even deeper than your thoughts and personality traits, and it's a bit of a mystery. It's the part of you that will go on living forever after your body dies. And if you are in Christ, it's the part of you that is instantly made new and one with the Holy Spirit when you believe. Because of this, God sees you like He sees Jesus: perfect, pure, and beloved. He is not angry at you, and never will be, because to Him you are His son or daughter, blameless and righteous. To be mad at you God would have to be mad at Jesus. Your spirit is the part of you that longs to commune with God, to be near Him, and to know Him more. It is the part of you that loves and desires good.

The Holy Spirit is continually working in your spirit to remind you of God's goodness and your righteousness by faith. He is leading you and "helping" you to see the truth and to make everyday decisions.

The Passion translation of John 16 calls the Holy Spirit the Divine Encourager. I love that!

The Holy Spirit is not here to continually convict you of your sin and condemn you if you're a believer of Christ. He is here to encourage you and remind you of who you are. Jesus tells us that the Spirit comes to convict the *world* of their sin because they do not believe in Him. If the Spirit is convicting people who do not believe in Jesus then He is convicting UNbelievers of their sin in order to point them to their need for a savior. Nowhere does Jesus tell us that the Spirit comes to keep condemning believers for their sin in order to make them feel ashamed. No, that comes from the devil, whose name means the "accuser".

Jesus goes on to say that the Spirit will convict us of our righteousness because when he went back to the father, we're no longer able to physically look upon Him. Finally, Jesus says the Spirit will convict the world of judgement because the ruler of this dark world has already been punished. In other words, the Spirit reminds us that Satan is the author of sin, and sin has already been judged and punished in Jesus' death on the cross. We are now free to stop punishing ourselves, and others, for sins that were already punished with Jesus.

And while the Spirit does not condemn us for our past sins, He does leads us down the right path, and He helps us to make the right decision and to step into God's plan for our lives. Sometimes this requires a big push in the opposite direction, sometimes it's found in the gentle nudges of our intuition.

If we do choose not to listen to His leading, then we disobey, and we step out of God's best for our lives. If we directly disobey direction from the Spirit we may deal with the natural consequences of not listening. Not because God is punishing us for our sin again and again, but because we didn't heed wise counsel. It's like this, let's say your boss wants to give you a surprise party and a promotion for how hard you've been working. He tells you to be at work tomorrow morning an hour early, and your coworkers text you that evening reminding you to set your alarm. If you decide to ignore them, you'd naturally miss out on the award, and maybe the promotion.

The Spirit's leading is similar. He works to encourage, equip, and prepare you for the future you can't see, but He can. He teaches you all things for your own good, even when you don't yet see why or how things are working out for your benefit. What's more, when we do mess up, God finds a way to take our mistakes and turn them around, He finds a way to get us back on the path for our good. He continues to bless us, because of His mercy and grace.

Ultimately, we are transformed when we listen and yield to the Spirit's direction. He will remind us of our identity in Christ. He will bring scripture to mind to help us in all situations. When we take the time to fill our minds with scripture, to pray and be silent before the Lord, and to listen to what the Spirit is telling us, then we begin to transform our thoughts, emotions, and desires (our soul) to align with what we're hearing and learning. As our soul transforms, parts of our personality may change for the better. We still remain uniquely us, as God designed us to be, but now we're becoming the best versions of ourselves, usually without consciously trying to change.

In the same way that we are not saved by cleaning up our act on the outside, we aren't transformed by focusing on good behaviors. Not to say that good behavior is a bad thing, but when we consciously seek to be good, to do better on our own, sin uses the opportunity of our stumbles to accuse and shame us. This brings me to the subject of the flesh.

FLESH: WHAT IT IS & WHAT IT ISN'T

Flesh. This term is the reason so many believers think the concept of listening to their body is sacrilege. They're bound and determined to believe that their body is evil, sinful, and untrustworthy. Why do they believe this? I think it's because they're confusing the usage of the term flesh in the Bible with our actual physical bodies. But when we look at the meaning of the word flesh in scripture it encompasses much more than skin and bones. Flesh refers to our entire being— spirit, soul, and body—working on its own, without the Lord.

In The Passion Translation, the word for flesh in Galatians 5:19 is literally translated "self-life." In other words, flesh is your desire for total control, self-effort, and self-glory. It's going out on your own and doing something of your own volition that is not guided or empowered by God. It's living for your own glory and recognition. Your flesh is the rebellious sin nature that believes God is holding out on you and urges you to take things into your own hands. Flesh is self-righteous; it will try to convince you that you can be good enough to earn God's respect and attention. It's also self-deprecating; it will remind you of your failures and tell you you'll never be good enough for God's love. Flesh is sneaky and sometimes disguises itself as good intentions. But any intention, and ultimately any action, done outside of faith in Jesus is sin and destined for failure.

Think of it this way: we know that God places desires in our heart that He wants to fulfill in our lives. Yet if we hasten to fulfill those desires on our own without Him (flesh), we'll likely end up hurt and disillusioned. Imagine the single woman who longs to be married and have children. If she waits on God, He is able to protect her and build her up until the right match comes along. If however, she takes matters into her own hands without being led by the spirit and starts throwing herself at every guy she meets, she will likely put herself through a lot of heartbreak and pain before she meets the man God intends for her.

Listen to what Paul says in Romans 7 about living in the flesh:

> For I know that nothing good dwells in me, that is, in my flesh. For I have the desire to do what is right, but not the ability to carry it out. For I do not do the good I want, but the evil I do not want is what I keep on doing. Now if I do what I do not want, it is no longer I who do it, but sin that dwells within me. Romans 7:18-20 ESV

So even when we desire to do the right thing and set out to do it, if we are led and empowered by our self-effort alone, then we end up doing the opposite. Our sin-nature seizes the opportunity of our flesh-directed efforts at doing good and causes a rebellion within us to rise.

The beautiful news of the gospel is that Jesus redeemed our entire being: spirit, soul, and body. So now, we no longer live by the flesh, by our self-led desires, but by the Spirit, who is perfect and good and all-knowing. You see, before Jesus died for our sins and gave us the Holy Spirit, people were left to try to follow the commandments on their own and earn righteousness by their own obedience and weak faith. But when Jesus came, He lived the perfect life, free from selfish pursuits and untainted by sin. He did what we could not. He had complete and total faith in the Father and His plan, a faith that surpassed anything we could muster on our own. Now, as the Father looks at us and sees us in

Christ, He sees Jesus' blameless life and great belief and calls us righteous, redeemed and full of faith. We are hidden in Christ when we believe in His all sufficient sacrifice.

Since all this is true, let's not waste time condemning our bodies as "sinful" when we know we are redeemed. Instead, let's remember that our bodies were created by a great God. He calls His design a masterpiece. When we listen to what our bodies are telling us, we listen to mechanisms designed and put in place by our creator for our good, and in doing this, we glorify Him and His creation.

Now, please don't misunderstand me. I am well aware that sometimes as believers we choose to live by the flesh, acting out of our own selfish desires, out of fear, mistrust in God's plan or maybe just out of an effort to go faster, harder, and do more. In these moments, we are hardly listening to our bodies. Usually we're ignoring them as a means to "get more done" or we're controlling them as a way to tame the chaos we feel from running ahead of God. Where food is concerned, this often manifests itself in one of a few ways: mindless overeating, undereating, low energy, dieting, eating disorders, or obsession.

So yes, when we are acting out of fear instead of faith, running ahead of God in the name of our own glory instead of His, pushing for busy instead of listening and relying on Him, we're rarely able to step back and care for our bodies in a God-honoring way—not because we can't trust our body's signals—but because we aren't trusting God enough to slow down and listen!

So how do we step into the total transformation that's already taken place in our Spirit? We stop insisting on fixing everything ourselves, and instead yield to the Holy

Spirit's work. We stop hustling for hustling's sake, and we get to know the wonder of our beautiful savior, Jesus, because He is the image of God.

And what about all those habits we already formed before we came to Jesus? What about our souls, many of them shaped by fallen people and experiences, and clouded by the distorted views of our society? What about those automatic thoughts that are contrary to God's Word? The ones that condemn us and call us back to guilt and striving for favor? That's what our sword is for. The sword is the Word of God and the Bible tells us that it is able to divide between spirit and soul (Hebrews 4:12). Meaning the Word of God will point out the truth that comes from the Holy Spirit and in contrast, it will expose the false beliefs we've been hanging onto in our soul. This will take place over and over again as we study God's Word and ask the Holy Spirit to teach us, until nothing false remains, until our souls are transformed into the image of Christ.

I hope you've figured out by now that God wants to use His Spirit to transform your entire being, spirit, soul, and body. This requires that we believe Him and His Word when He says He is good, and He alone is our deliverance and strength (Isaiah 45:24). Not self-denial, not food, not exercise, and not approval from man.

When we do this, when we place ourselves at Christ's feet and admit that He alone can do all things, then He's able to pick up the messy clay of our lives and shape it into a vessel for His glory and our joy! And wow, how infinitely better is that than the temporary high of posting a #transformationtuesday picture? Am I right?

REFLECTION QUESTIONS:

1. What fantasies have you had about being transformed? What area of your life do you most want God to transform? How can you give your transformation over to Him and let go of your self-led efforts?

2. Since becoming a Christian, have you witnessed any changes in yourself that you didn't instigate? How do you think God was involved?

3. What past beliefs, emotions, and thought patterns are you holding onto? How can you let the Spirit transform them?

4. What's one way that your body suffers when you're doing things on your own, without God, or going ahead of Him? What's something you could do to remedy this?

Chapter 7

NO POWER IN RESTRICTION & REGULATIONS

"…you died with Christ to the elemental spiritual forces of this world, why, as though you still belonged to the world, do you submit to its rules: 'Do not handle! Do not taste! Do not touch!'? These rules, which have to do with things that are all destined to perish with use, are based on merely human commands and teachings. Such regulations indeed have an appearance of wisdom, with their self-imposed worship, their false humility and their harsh treatment of the body, but they lack any value in restraining sensual indulgence."

COLOSSIANS 2:20-23 NIV

RESTRICTION & RUMINATION

Have you ever tried to "quit" something cold turkey? Maybe you tried to quit smoking, nail biting, or eating sweets. Do you remember how hard it was? Were you successful long term? And if so, was it all on your own or was God captaining the ship?

I surveyed my friends and followers on social media and asked an initial question and a follow up questions:

- What are you actively trying to stop doing?
- Has focusing on quitting made it harder or easier?

Among the people who responded, I got answers about trying to:

- Quit mindlessly scrolling through social media
- Stop biting my nails
- Quit bingeing on food in the evening
- Stop counting calories

My follow up question revealed every single person observed focusing on quitting a behavior had made it harder to stop, not easier.

I was completely unsurprised by these results because they confirmed my suspicions about human nature and solidified what scripture and the scientific research say about restriction.

We know from experience that the mindset of restriction and physical deprivation actually intensifies our desire for the very thing we're restricting. Think about the garden of Eden and the term forbidden fruit. Our flesh wants what we tell ourselves we can't have. We call the continual, obsessive thoughts that result from focusing on restriction, rumination. I love this word, because it paints a perfect picture. One of the definitions of ruminate means to chew repeatedly, and sometimes as is the case with cows, it means chewing, swallowing, regurgitating, and then continuing to chew.

When we ruminate on a thought, the thought refuses to disappear. Instead it is regurgitated at every opportunity. If you've ever suffered from fear or anxiety, you likely know what I'm talking about. Maybe you've gone to bed at night and repeatedly played out the same scenario, analyzing it from every angle until you feel physically ill. Restriction can have this sort of effect. And when it comes to eliminating foods, the more physically deprived we are, the worse we ruminate about food.

Of course, we aren't all restricting big quantities of energy, but the brain is a powerful thing. Even the thought of cutting out a food will increase our desire for it. The best way I can think to explain this phenomenon is with a story about dieting.

I once attempted to fast from (give up) all added sugar for a month. And before you think I was all super spiritual and led by God to do this, I was not sitting in quiet time pouring out my heart to God, listening for His voice when I decided to restrict. Nope, this decision of mine was all self-directed and purely motivated by a desire to change my body's appearance and cope with the new anxieties of being a mom. Flash forward to the days before the sugar fast began. My brain, being fully aware of the upcoming restriction, amped up the signals for sweets. Thoughts like, you better get all the cookies you can now, because in a few days it's sayonara, drove me to eat way more sweets than normal, and this was all before I started restricting sugar. Of course, this only made me more convinced of my "addiction" to sweets and my need to restrict them. As the day rolled around, I began actively avoiding things with added sugar in them. And it worked—well sort of, for a time.

I lost a little weight and my clothes fit a little differently—likely due to the dehydrating effects of lower carb diets. And if I'm being honest, I felt proud, accomplished, and self-righteous. Look at me, high on my dietitian horse: I'm smart, I'm researched, I have the answers—HA!

Despite this, my brain began dutifully urging me to eat sugar, quietly at first and then loudly. By the end of 2 weeks, my cravings for sweets were at an all-time high! And my new mom anxieties and mood swings? They weren't any better; actually, the stress of restricting sugar sent me into high anxiety and even bigger emotional dips than before. At some point, I gave in and ate some sweets. After that, the all-or-nothing thinking took over. You already ate some sugar, might as well have another donut and a candy bar and while we're at it, everything else that's sweet. Let's have that too! After the all-out eating followed the accusations: You have no self-control. How can you call yourself a dietitian if you can't even do this one thing? How do you expect to be a good mom if you can't control yourself? Then they got worse: You've asked God to help you lose weight and He isn't helping you, He's most likely mad at you, that's why He isn't listening.

The devil is a cunning liar. He doesn't come right out and call you unworthy and unloved by God. No, he builds up to it, he uses our weaknesses, the areas where we're trying to forge ahead alone, to accuse us. He points to our failures and calls them God's fault. And then he makes us question God's goodness, our salvation, and the reality of grace.

IT'S IN OUR NATURE

It is our nature to rebel against rules and restrictions. Think about any toddler, or any teenager, you've been around (even if it was you). When we tell kids not to do something, the majority of the time they go out of their way to do that very thing.

Not too long ago my sister tested this theory. She looked at my two-year-old, who was contentedly playing in the kitchen, and said, "Judah, don't go play in the living room." All the sudden, my previously happy child started pouting and whining about the living room until he finally walked himself over to the living room and just stood there and looked guilty. No, I don't suggest you invoke this sort of cruel behavior on your kids. My family is just a bunch of practical jokers. In all seriousness, for many parents the solution to this natural rebellion is to punish, punish, punish. "Effective" punishment results in the child being afraid to misbehave—at least for a time. Eventually, when their parents aren't around, and the threat of punishment is gone, most kids will do the forbidden thing anyway, and then shame will enter in to point out their failure.

It's been this way from the beginning, ever since Adam and Eve first ate from the tree. God knows this; He knows our weak human tendencies. That's why He sent Jesus to do what we could not do, and that's why He gives us the Holy Spirit to enable and empower us to live the life He's called us to. He knows there is no power in rules or self-denial to make us better. The power lies with Him and His perfect love—and perfect love drives out fear, because fear implies punishment (1 John 4:18), but there is no more punishment for those who believe; every sin was already punished on the cross of Jesus Christ (Romans 3:21-31).

You see, even though we ask for God's help avoiding certain foods, with dieting or weight loss, it doesn't mean these are good things or God things, and it doesn't mean your efforts will suddenly be productive. The entire point of following Jesus is not to ask Him to bless OUR will, but to seek out HIS will first and then follow it confidently, knowing it will lead to our good and His glory.

And His will for us is not to focus on restriction, self-denial, or religion. He asks us to focus on Him and His grace, love, and all-sufficiency.

Paul wrote to the church at Colossae concerning their trust in religious systems and physical deprivation for righteousness, urging them to remember that they already died to that way of life:

> For you were included in the death of Christ and have died with Him to the religious system and powers of this world. Don't retreat back to being bullied by the standards and opinions of religion— for example, their strict requirements, "You can't associate with that person!" or, "Don't eat that!" or, "You can't touch that!" These are the doctrines of men and corrupt customs that are worthless to help you spiritually. Colossians 2: 20 – 22 TPT

The Colossians, like many Christians today, were attempting to return to the Law after receiving the gospel of grace. Apparently, some religious teachers were trying to convince them of their need to follow regulations and customs of restriction, "don't taste, don't touch." But Paul very clearly warns the Colossians not to associate with such people, assuring them that these man-made doctrines and customs were worthless to help them spiritually.

In the same way, dietary rules and regulations are worthless to help us in spirit today. We know it is the Holy Spirit within us that renews all things and transforms us, so it benefits us to focus on the two things that do help us spiritually—the gospel of God's grace through Jesus Christ and the Holy Spirit's guidance.

Paul goes on to write that though these people promoting restriction have the appearance of wisdom, when they engage in deprivation of their physical bodies their actions are rooted in nothing more than religious activity!

I think it's easy to write passages like these off, claiming they were written for another time and a different culture. But scripture hasn't been kept around and meticulously maintained for thousands of years only to be relevant to a past generation. The Word of God is alive and applicable today.

And honestly, we might as well be living among the Colossians now. Think about all the programs rooted in restriction and physical deprivation, think about the people behind them who claim to have the answers to health, life, and happiness. We're fascinated with things like fasting, veganism, and keto diets. All of which point to restriction as the answer to all of our ailments. We've started adopting more and more extreme forms of exercise like ultra-marathons, extreme obstacle races, Ironman, and CrossFit. I don't point these out because there's anything inherently wrong with them, but rather to demonstrate the cultural trend towards restriction and pushing our bodies to greater and greater heights.

And why? Why are we subjecting ourselves to it all? For many of us, we've believed the lie that deprivation is good, that it makes us a better person, and healthier to boot! After all, how can we expect to be healthy, happy, and fulfilled if we don't do something extremely sacrificial to earn it? No matter how much we claim to believe in grace, we have a really hard time letting it seep into every area of our lives. The whole thing just doesn't fit with our concept of fairness. Yet, if we take the Word at face value, then we know that God doesn't see our sins, instead He sees us as a beloved child. And a good father who loves His children dearly doesn't need a reason to bless them with good things, He just does. It's the same with our heavenly father.

God already calls you redeemed, He already loves you like a daughter or a son, and apart from asking, you don't need to do anything on your own in order to receive good gifts from Him. Nothing you did was good enough to earn justification, and nothing you do will be good enough to earn blessings and favor. It's all undeserved, yet freely given, it's all grace.

The idea that physical restriction is the answer to our physical health is not unlike the idea that never spending money is the answer to financial security and happiness. On the surface it appears like a wise decision to be a cheapskate, but when you live your whole life saying no to everything, hoarding your money, you miss out on the opportunity to experience life, to give to others, and to invest wisely. Like

Charles Dickens's Ebenezer Scrooge, we can become cold and calculated, isolating ourselves from the rest of the world. When you decide on your own to start cutting out foods from your diet and forcing yourself to go to the gym, does it bring you closer to God? Closer to those around you? More than likely these types of behaviors only serve to make you more preoccupied with food, exercise, and your body, leaving you with very little time and energy for seeking God and loving others.

FREEDOM & EMPOWERMENT IN CHRIST

In Christ we've been set free from this struggle. It's my hope that we don't submit again to bondage, to the religious laws and regulations that promote restriction and sacrifice above mercy and grace. If our motivation for eating is rooted in trying to earn worthiness, acceptance, or salvation, we're going back to the old way of doing things.

Before Jesus died and rose and made us righteous by grace through faith, our only hope for salvation was in following the Law. And not just the Ten Commandments, but the countless ceremonial and handling laws, laws about how to eat, and laws defining clean and unclean foods.

Spoiler alert, no one has ever done this perfectly, except for Jesus. He came to fulfil the law given by Moses so that we can live by a higher standard of faith in Him and cease being enslaved to our sin nature.

Just like restriction naturally results in an obsessive desire for the thing or behavior being restricted, attempts to follow the law, to be good, while well-intended, awaken the sinful, rebellious nature within us and ultimately cause us to do the thing we're trying not to do.

Read Galatians 3:9–14. We know we are not made righteous by keeping the law, but by faith. And keeping the law does not require faith, but self-directed effort. In his letter to the Galatians, Paul urges believers not to return to the legalistic bondage of the law, for anyone who does this is effectively putting themselves back under sin's curse. And if we choose to practice the law we must follow ALL of the Law, which includes all 613 rules and regulations recorded by Moses in the Old Testament! I don't know about you, but I've tried being a perfect rule follower and God knows I'm no match for it. Thank God for Jesus and his covering of my shortcomings.

Does this mean we should just keep sinning, recklessly hurting everyone in our path? Of course not. When we cling to grace we are not making light of evil's terrible stench, but instead we are making much of Jesus' all sufficient, life, death, resurrection, and indwelling in us. And the more we make of Jesus and His empowering grace, the less we focus on ourselves and our power.

Eating food is not sinful, neither is food morally bad or unclean. Jesus redeemed all foods when He declared that nothing that enters a man from the outside defiles him (Mark 7:15). Yet, when we impose rules over our lives about what we can and can't eat, when we label ourselves good for eating one way and bad for eating another, we're nullifying the word of Christ and the grace of God in our consciences. Beyond that, we respond to these self-directed restrictions in the same way we respond to efforts to behave by following the law—with rebellion. As Paul says in Romans 7, "we do what we do not want to do."

Do you want to know what one of the biggest predictors of weight gain, binge-eating, and disordered eating is? It's food restriction. Regardless of the form, restricting whole food groups, calories, carbs, fat, or protein does not work in the long term.[1] Further, dieting has been shown to increase chronic psychological stress and cortisol production.[1] So not only is self-directed dietary restriction unhelpful for lasting transformation, it may even cause undesirable side effects. Further, we miss out on important nutrients and increase rates of mortality when we eliminate just one food group, like whole grains, [2] not to mention forms of eating that require the elimination of *several* food groups.

God is able to sustain you through all things, but why submit to all that physical and mental stress when you could be free AND healthy living another way?

Jesus gave us the solution to our struggles with restriction and failure, and our inability to follow the Law, He supplies us with the answer in Himself. He is the bread of life, which means that He sustains us, provides for us, and upholds us in health. We look to His life and ministry and we see that He did nothing of His own accord (flesh), but only what the father told Him to do. We are called to do the same.

And let me tell you, the father is not calling you to a life of slavery to food rules or religious standards, but to a life of listening to His still, small voice. A voice that isn't angry with you, a voice that doesn't condemn, shame, or berate you. His voice always guides you forward in love, sending you "gut instincts" about all things, revealing the hidden meaning of scripture and grace to you like never before. This is the voice of God, His Holy Spirit in you and He is faithful to lead you into all good things. So, trust him, not dieting, not rules and regulations, and not the world— trust Jesus.

REFLECTION QUESTIONS:

1. What have you tried quit or restrict apart from God, how did that turn out? Did you find yourself feeling empowered or drawn to doing what you did not want to do?

2. How does the knowledge that you are dead to the Law set you free to trust Jesus? Are you ruminating on sin or striving to earn God's blessing? What can you let go of?

3. What's your experience with restricting food? Did it make you feel closer to or further away from God?

4. Have you ever thought of your gut instinct or intuition as separate from your mind? Do you pay attention to your gut? What, if anything, has it been telling you lately?

Chapter 8

KNOW THAT ALL FOODS FIT

"Now the Spirit expressly says that in later times some will depart from the faith by devoting themselves to deceitful spirits and teachings of demons, through the insincerity of liars whose consciences are seared, who forbid marriage and require abstinence from foods that God created to be received with thanksgiving by those who believe and know the truth. For everything created by God is good, and nothing is to be rejected if it is received with thanksgiving, for it is made holy by the word of God and prayer."

1 TIMOTHY 4:1-5 ESV

I once watched a 3-minute video clip from FunnyorDie.com called "Time Traveling Dietitian"—if you haven't seen it yet, go watch it[1]! It's hilarious, but it's also so scary accurate that it stings. The premise is this: a time-traveling dietitian from the future visits a couple from 1979 during their breakfast. The wife is just getting ready to hand her husband a plate of steak and eggs with toast and butter. During his first visit, the dietitian warns the couple about the harmful effects of dietary cholesterol stating that "even one egg could kill you," and then disappearing back to the future. Out of a loving concern for her husband, the wife quickly takes his plate to throw away the eggs, within seconds the time traveling dietitian is back. This time he claims that it's only the yolks that need to be avoided and then disappears again, but the wife has already thrown away her husband's eggs.

The third time he returns, the dietitian admits that eggs are actually fine, and that dietary cholesterol doesn't affect blood cholesterol, saying "We actually aren't even sure what cholesterol does." But before he disappears again, he passionately warns against eating red meat, claiming it causes heart disease. The husband starts to get visibly annoyed at this point and as his wife goes to throw away his steak, he tells her to wait. Sure enough, the time traveling dietitian comes back again stating that steak is fine, but that man was never meant to eat bread. This time the couple is a little more suspicious of his recommendations. He claims they're based on what our "Paleolithic ancestors ate" but can't be sure because it's just a guess.

The wife urges the dietitian to visit the Paleolithic era and verify what they're eating. Hilariously, the dietitian returns, his clothes all torn up and his glasses askew. His words to the couple, "They are NOT doing well back there, if anything we should all be eating a whole lot more bread." "Just eat what you want and exercise," he says.

Now, obviously this is a fictional skit, but it reflects the way many feel about food in our culture: fearful and confused. The science of nutrition is relatively young, and as such, it's constantly changing. We're making new discoveries every day, and many of the things we thought we understood at first (i.e. dietary cholesterol causing heart disease) are now claims we're having to correct.

The problem is we get so caught up in the latest nutrient or latest food fad, and we immediately label them good, as with turmeric, kale, and omega-3s, or we demonize them as evil. In the past we've deemed saturated fat, eggs, and red meat as bad. Today, all of these are suddenly good again! And now the foods we used to think of as good: grains, dairy, fruit, and carbohydrates in general are now being called junk.

Can't you see the hypocrisy of it all? Nutrition is not a black and white science, and we don't understand everything about food yet, not even close. However, even with our incomplete knowledge, we've managed to overcomplicate eating so much that the majority of people are confused about what to eat. And when you boil down all the confusion, everyone is asking some variation of the same question: what's good for me to eat and what's bad for me to eat?

Here's a radical thought: food isn't good or bad. It's neither clean nor unclean. It's not pure, nor is it junk——food is food. Yes, some foods are more nutrient dense. Some foods taste delicious and some foods taste like cardboard. Some foods are satisfying and some foods leave us wanting. Some foods are hot, some foods are cold, some are sour, some are sweet, and some I really like to eat. The point is that food is not morally good or bad. It's just food.

Every food has something to offer someone in one situation or another. For instance, you might think Cheetos are the worst food imaginable (exaggerating on purpose here). But somebody else who lives in an impoverished area, and whose only option is a bag of Cheetos at the local convenience store, is probably pretty happy about the energy and enjoyment those Cheetos provide.

When we demonize certain foods, and glorify others, we make people who aren't of the same socioeconomic standing feel guilty for eating the only foods they have access to. We make families feel inadequate for feeding their loved-ones traditional foods that have kept them alive and happy for years, foods they know, foods they can afford.

If this doesn't stir up something in us, then let's look to the effects of labeling foods good or bad on our own mental and physical well-being. Whether we realize it or not, classifying food as good or bad sets us up to feel pretty terrible about ourselves. Because ultimately one of three things will happen:

- Option one: We'll give into eating our "bad" foods because of a thought like "I deserve it, I've had a bad day," or "I've been good all week," but due to the increased desire that comes with restricting foods, we'll way overdo it, leaving us in a heap of shame.

- Option two: In a situation we have no control over, the only choice will be to eat a "bad" food, so we'll do it. But because we feel guilty about eating, we'll either compensate by punishing ourselves with exercise, more restriction or purging, or we'll revert to the good old, what-the-heck, might-as-well-eat-it-all-for-the-next-week mentality.

- Option three: We'll isolate ourselves from situations where we can't control the food options. In which case, our relationships will tend to suffer and we'll either start believing the lies that we're unlovable, or better yet, we'll feel self-righteous for our great sacrifices in the name of eating "clean."

None of these options are pretty, and none of them are healthy. True health encompasses much more than diet and exercise, it involves psychological, relational, emotional, and spiritual aspects of well-being. If eating good foods and avoiding bad foods takes away from any of these areas, if it steals your peace, then it's not healthy for you.

If moralizing food results in all of this shame and turmoil, it only makes sense that we STOP doing it. Amen?

Instead of judging food as good or bad, clean or unclean, right or wrong, or any variation of these, let's describe it for its beneficial qualities. I like to think of this as the "lovely food" principle.

In his letter to the Philippians, the apostle Paul writes:

> Finally, brothers and sisters, whatever is true, whatever is noble, whatever is right, whatever is pure, whatever is lovely, whatever is admirable—if anything is excellent or praiseworthy—think about such things. Whatever you have learned or received or heard from me or seen in me—put it into practice. And the God of peace will be with you. Philippians 4:8-9 NIV

I think we can apply these words to food. Every food has something lovely about it, something to be grateful for—even if it doesn't contain the latest buzz-worthy-nutrient.

It could be that you're thankful for your grandmother's apple pie because it reminds you of sweet family memories or because it fills you up, gives you energy, and satisfies you until the next meal. Or maybe you had a tub of movie theatre popcorn and you recall that it was salty and delicious. The apple you had while working in your garden was refreshing, sweet, and satisfying. That bag of Doritos your mother-in-law gave you in the car helped hold you over and keep your energy levels steady until you could get home for lunch.

Even if you don't feel like speaking positively about the food you're eating, making the shift from moral adjectives to objective, neutral descriptors is a powerful step towards removing the stigma and fear around food. Using words like hot, cold, warm, soft, hydrating, crunchy, sweet, rich, and filling is a more accurate way to describe food and is much less damaging than labeling food good and bad.

Ultimately, what we're doing when we shift the way we talk about food is refusing to pass moral judgement on ourselves and others for individual food choices. And while language is important and powerful, the real transformation happens in our changing beliefs about food. There's a concept in psychology called cognitive dissonance, wherein we purposely say something out loud that is contrary to what we believe. It looks like this: if I believe I am worthless, then every time I have those thoughts, I would say out loud the opposite, maybe, "I am worthy to be loved because Jesus died for me." Eventually, if we keep speaking in the way that we would like to believe, and meditating on it, our brain will follow suit. It can be the same with food. If we continue to use our words to objectively and positively describe all foods about their positive or neutral qualities, our mind will eventually agree.

But even more than employing cognitive dissonance, we as Christians are encouraged to demolish every argument and stronghold that sets itself up against the knowledge of God. We're called to take every thought captive and make it obedient to Christ's truth (2 Corinthians 10: 5). So, let's use our spiritual weapon, the word of God to do that with food.

The Bible is very clear. Jesus redeemed all foods. He made all food clean and good for us to eat. We are no longer called to observe dietary laws and restrictions, as was true under the old covenant. But don't take my word for it. God addressed this issue (yes, he even addresses food) in the New Testament.

In Mark 7:15 and Matthew 15:11 Jesus said that nothing that enters a man defiles him, only that which comes out of his mouth from his heart defiles him. With these words He made all food clean and also pointed to the importance of our heart and the belief or unbelief we hold there. Jesus knew that eventually, what's in a man's heart will exit his mouth and will either profess faith to salvation or unbelief which harms him (Romans 10:9-10, Proverbs 4:23, Proverbs 10:11).

In Matthew 5:17 Jesus said that he did not come to abolish the law of Moses (which included dietary restrictions), but rather to bring it to fulfillment, or completion, and accomplish its purpose once and for all.

Paul tells us that the purpose of the law was temporary, for a short time in history it made the Jewish people more aware of their sin, pointing them more and more to their need for a savior, until the one who was promised (Jesus) arrived (Galatians 3:19–25). When He came, Jesus fulfilled the requirements of the law. The law's purpose has been accomplished in us already if we believed in Christ and is still being accomplished in non-believers as it points people to their need for Jesus. Once we accept the truth that we cannot fulfil the law on our own and believe that all of our sins were punished on Jesus, we are justified and we enter into the NEW covenant, the one God promised to make with His people in Jeremiah 31:31. This new covenant is not dependent on following the law of Moses, but it is dependent on our faith in Jesus and God's grace (Galatians 3). We now live by a higher law, the law of love which is placed inside of us when we believe. This perfect love is also the fruit produced in us, not by our own efforts, but by the Holy Spirit's working in us (Galatians 5:22).

In Acts 10:9-16 God gave Peter a vision of previously unclean animals coming down from heaven and told him to arise, kill, and eat. When Peter protested eating food that was prohibited in the law of Moses, God told Peter not to call anything impure that He had made clean. Soon after, Peter was called to go into the house of a gentile, eat with him and his family, and ultimately, bring them the gospel. Before the new covenant of Christ, spanning from the time of Moses to Jesus (about 1500 years), the Jewish people were prohibited from eating certain foods, foods that the gentiles (non-Jewish people) would have eaten. In fact, it was looked upon as unclean to even eat at the same table as a gentile. If God had not redeemed all food through Christ and reminded Peter of this in a vision, then Peter likely never would have brought the gospel to that non-Jewish household.

Paul addressed the topic of food several times throughout his letters to the churches, but arguably the best passage in favor of food freedom comes in one of his letters to Timothy. In the letter he warns Timothy about the "doctrines of demons" that will be taught in the last days. And what does he say these doctrines will teach? Well to the surprise of many, the false prophets of the last days won't be teaching licentiousness and condoning sins, they won't be urging people to keep on with their bad habits because it's okay. No, Paul says that these people will teach others to abstain from marriage and from foods that God has made to be received by those who know the truth, the truth of the gospel of grace. He goes on to say that all foods, and everything created by God is good and nothing is to be rejected if received with thanksgiving (1 Timothy 4:5).

It just doesn't get any clearer than that. There is no power in food to make us good or bad. Only Jesus redeems us, and what he's called clean we shouldn't speak of as impure—that includes us too.

C.S. Lewis talked about this in his book *Mere Christianity* when he wrote:

> An individual christian may see fit to give up all sort s of things for special reasons—marriage, or meat, or beer, or cinema; but the moment he starts saying the things are in themselves bad, or looking down his

nose at other people who do use them, he has taken the wrong turning.

We know that there is freedom in Christ, as individuals, to eat as we are led, exercise as we are led, and generally live as we are led, as long as what we do is for the glory of God and does not expressly contradict the teachings of Christ. As such, we are not called to judge another person's eating nor are we called to question what God is calling them to do or not do (unless a fellow believer comes to us for advice and what they're doing goes against the knowledge of Christ).

Each of us is called to run our own race and to fulfill God's purposes for our lives. We do this by getting to know Him, by listening to the Holy Spirit's stirrings in us, and by taking steps of faith to obey those things that He's calling us to.

The beauty of the grace filled life is that we are not accountable to man, but to God, and God alone. As a result, we are free to listen to Him without comparing our journey to someone else's or submitting to another person's convictions. Effectively, this gives us the right to choose what we want to eat and how we want to move our bodies based on our personal preferences, convictions, and lifestyle.

Don't give up your freedom in this area in order to submit to somebody else's convictions, instead allow God to lead you personally in all things. Similarly, just because you've found that avoiding certain foods is beneficial for you, it doesn't give you the right to impose your convictions on another believer or the right to judge them for not eating the way you do.

Paul writes about this very subject in Romans 14:1-4 ESV.

> As for the one who is weak in faith, welcome him, but not to quarrel over opinions. One person believes he may eat anything, while the weak person eats only vegetables. Let not the one who eats despise the one who abstains and let not the one who abstains pass judgment on the one who eats, for God has welcomed him. Who are you to pass judgment on the servant of another? It is before his own master that he stands or falls. And he will be upheld, for the Lord is able to make him stand.

He goes on to explain that each believer who is led by a personal conviction from God about matters of eating or drinking does it to honor the Lord and also gives thanks to God.

The key here, is that the motivation for eating or not eating comes from a personal conviction and is done to honor and give thanks to God. Notice Paul did not say that eating or avoiding certain foods should be used to acquire peace or to manipulate or punish our bodies. He didn't say restricting certain foods was holier or that it was necessary for a well-lived life.

Actually, he goes on to write,

> I know and am convinced by personal revelation from the Lord Jesus that there is nothing wrong with

eating any food. But to the one who considers it to be unclean, it is unacceptable. Romans 14:14 TPT.

This goes back to the concept of maintaining a grace-focused conscience instead of one focused on guilt, so we don't give way to condemnation and shame. If you, in your conscience, feel guilty about eating certain foods, then in order to maintain a peaceful conscience you'll have to avoid them. But wouldn't it be so much better altogether if we made peace with food? If we all believed, like Paul, that there is nothing wrong with eating any food? Then, we wouldn't have to struggle with avoiding certain foods and the resultant guilt over eating them.

It's nearly impossible to listen to your intuition, to the Spirit, if your conscience is clouded with guilt. It's hard to make decisions based on what's best for your body when you still fear food. For this reason, it's imperative that we make peace with the foods we've been calling "bad." When we do, food loses its power over us, clearing our conscience so that all we hear is God leading us through His Spirit and our intuition.

OVERCOMING FEAR FOODS

Up until this point in the book, we've focused on aligning our beliefs about ourselves, God, and food with the knowledge of grace. If you're still feeling very fearful of foods, I encourage you to go back and work through those chapters some more, meditating on the scriptures we talked about. If you're feeling less anxious and ready to move forward, we're going to take action to make peace with food.

Get out your pen and paper and make a list of ten foods you love, but maybe try to avoid because you've thought of them as bad. If you've been under the impression that you're "addicted" to any foods, write these foods down now. Depending on how you feel, go stock your house with one to three of the food items on your list. You can start with the foods that make you a little less anxious and work your way to the more difficult ones.

Now you're going to do the thing; you're going to eat the foods. Set yourself up for success. That means when you eat the foods, make sure you aren't ravenous, that you haven't skipped meals, or restricted calories. Make yourself a regular snack or meal and include your challenge food. Eat it mindfully, savor the flavor, and refrain from judging yourself or the food.

How does it taste, smell, and feel in your mouth? Notice if it continues to taste great the entire time you're eating it or if it starts to lose its flavor. When you begin to feel comfortably full, stop eating. If you feel anxious afterwards, don't compensate by restricting or exercising, instead pray, thank God for the food and meditate on the truth of Christ's all-sufficient work. Now keep doing this, meal after meal, day after day with the same exact food. Each time you become full, remind yourself that you can have that food anytime you want it. Keep it stocked in your house. Do this until the food either becomes less appealing to you, as in you no longer crave it, or until you no longer feel out of control or anxious about eating it. Congratulations, that food no longer has power over you. You can choose to enjoy it whenever you want.

Move from one fear food to the next until you have made peace with every food or until you no longer feel anxious about eating. For the majority of people, it only takes challenging a few foods before they reach a place of peace with all food. The more consistent you are with eating the same exact food (i.e. same flavor and brand of ice cream, pizza, etc.) the quicker you'll be able to come to peace with it. And don't worry about nutrient deficiencies. Even if you ate the same food for three weeks, you're also eating other foods with it. Your body WILL get the nutrients it needs and tell you when to stop eating. Your God will sustain you.

FOOD ADDICTION

Working through this process can seem counterintuitive to those who view their struggles with food as an addiction. Often, self-proclaimed "food addicts" feel that they have to keep certain foods completely out of site and out of mind. Several of my clients have told me that eating even one bite of certain foods is likely to send them into a full-blown binge, which will only end when they gain 100 lbs. (or some variation of this fear). But we now know the truth that restricting foods, and calling them good and bad, is actually what sets us up to feel out of control around food. Besides that, there are many of us who would argue that when you look at the research, the entire concept of food addiction comes into question.

Many people will cite studies that state that sugar is addictive because it activates the reward centers of our brain. But what these studies show is that *restriction* and *semi starvation* cause the reward center in the brain to light up in response to eating sugar.[2] Eating carbohydrates (sugar) is essential for survival. Our body's role is to keep us healthy, and when it senses that we're actively restricting or contemplating restricting an essential nutrient, like sugar, it kicks into gear. The response is an increased desire for the restricted food. This maintains our drive to eat and eating keeps us alive! Just because eating sugar causes the release of happy neurotransmitters in our brain does not make it equivalent to a drug, it simply means our brain has been designed to keep us alive.

When you have a craving for a food you believe you're addicted to—let's say sweets—only the specific sweet you're craving will satisfy, and usually it's a treat you view as bad. If you were really addicted to sugar, then any sugar rich food would do the trick—something like a banana or a spoonful of plain sugar, let's say. But most people, if they try to meet their craving for gummy worms with a banana, will not be satisfied. You might argue that it's not sugar, but the highly palatable combination of fat and sugar that's addictive. But even still, if you're really craving a cookie and eat whole grain macaroni and cheese instead (another food with fat and sugar) you still won't be completely satisfied.

Although we certainly have research that questions the validity of the food addiction model, [2] maybe the best argument I have against it is my clinical experience.

Sam and Darla came to see me after trying every diet known to man. They were ready to stop throwing away money and willing to let go of dieting for the sake of their and their children's health. Sam told me on his first appointment that he was addicted to fast food. Darla had similar reservations about ice cream. We worked to remove the good and bad food labels and to give them unconditional permission to eat all foods, including fast food and ice cream. After doing this, Darla told me in session that ice cream had become less appealing, she sometimes ate it, but didn't find herself drawn to it like before. Similarly, Sam admitted that he no longer felt addicted to fast food, but ate it on occasion, when he wanted it, and stopped eating when full. This happens all of the time in my practice. When clients learn to fuel themselves regularly, when they stop restricting food, and stop viewing food as bad or good, the addictive power of foods goes away.

Contrary to true chemical dependence, like drug and alcohol addiction, the best way to eliminate "food addictions" is exposure. The more you allow yourself to mindfully enjoy all foods in a relaxed state and calm environment, the less out of control you'll feel. Positive food experiences matter. By eliminating good and bad food labels and allowing ourselves to eat all foods, we're creating trust in our relationship with food and body, and this trust empowers us to nourish our bodies the way that they need.

REFLECTION QUESTIONS

1. How are you attaching good and bad labels to food? How has this caused you too feel worse around food? How has it served you?

2. How can you change the way you talk about food so that you're able to enjoy it and align your thoughts with scripture?

3. List 5-10 or your favorite foods. Circle the ones you've been avoiding because you see it as bad or unhealthy. How can you challenge those feelings towards that food? Make a food exposure plan.

4. Are there any foods you feel addicted to? Ask God to reveal the truth about these to you. Do you have any deeper moral beliefs about those foods and what they'll do to you?

Chapter 9

THE GIFT OF WISE DISCRETION FOR EATING

"For God will never give you the spirit of fear, but the Holy Spirit who gives you mighty power, love, and self-control (revelation-light, instruction)."

2 TIMOTHY 1:7 TPT

YOU HAVE A GIFT, BUT YOU'RE USING IT ALL WRONG

Self-control. It's a concept I'm continually trying to teach my 2-year-old. "Pease, love the doggy, don't jump on him, honey." or "Poop, goes in the potty, not on the floor." We've had to teach him to stay in his bed at night, wait patiently at the check-out line as the clerk rings up his toy, and to ask for help when he's frustrated, instead of throwing a fit. We're teaching him all of these things so that he won't cause harm to himself or others. Ok, poop on the floor might not cause anyone serious harm right now, but eventually it's going to cause somebody emotional harm if a ten-year-old boy is still pooping on the floor. But you get the point, we're teaching him to control his impulses and make wise decisions for his own good and the good of others. We even have this little daily affirmation that he says, "I choose wisely."

As adults, we tend to think of self-control as the ability to stop ourselves from acting on our physical impulses, period. But is that really wise? If you're feeling ill would you ignore this feeling or would you see a doctor? If you have to go to the bathroom is it wise to just suppress this? Wouldn't you seek to find a bathroom as soon as possible? The Greek term *sōphronismou* in 2 Timothy 1:7 is translated as self-control. Self-control in English means revelation-light, instruction, wise-discretion.[1,2] It doesn't mean restriction, deprivation, or self-directed effort, but those are the meanings we've ascribed to it today.

In the world of health and fitness we've blamed our "poor" self-control for why we can't follow restrictive diets or rigorous workout plans. But do these things fit with our definition of self-control as wise-discretion? Is it wise to restrict food groups and calories throughout the day based off an arbitrary calculation? Scientifically speaking, no. That's a diet, and diets fail us in the long run, causing weight regain, slower metabolisms, central fat accumulation, increased fear of food, and lower self-confidence.[3] Spiritually, we know that self-imposed restriction has no power for blessing or transformation. Further, when we will-power our way to restricting food or food groups we increase the risk of bingeing.

So many people who struggle with bingeing or binge/ purge eating disorders are convinced the problem lies within them and their poor self-control. More times than not, bingeing is related to some form of restriction, whether from food rules, calorie deficits, or anticipated restriction (i.e.

planning to diet the next day). Our bodies are smart; when they sense restriction coming they amp up the signals to binge.

On the flip side, using self-discipline to engage in constant strenuous physical activity, despite your body's plea for rest or easier movement, leads to burnout at best and serious injury at worst. Yet we know from 2 Timothy 1:7 that the Holy Spirit has given us this gift of self-control or wise-discretion. We have it. So maybe it's not that we're lacking in this area, but rather that we're using our gift all wrong.

Self-control means being able to make a wise choice for our good and the good of others. But who defines what is wise and beneficial and what is not? God does. He is the giver of all wisdom and He alone can tell us what to do because He's the only one who knows us fully. He knows what our future holds and the safest route to get there. If it were up to us to determine what was beneficial, we'd be justifying every juice cleanse, relationship, and Netflix binge. And maybe those things are okay for you, but you won't know unless you listen to the guiding voice of your father, through the Holy Spirit, the one who gives us instruction.

Just like my son learns what decisions are wise and which are unwise from his parents, we also lean on our father to give us direction. And as parents we don't raise every child the same because each one is unique. Our heavenly Father does the same with His children. He may give you different instructions than your sister. That doesn't make you right and her wrong, it just means God knows what you need better than you do. He knows you each are on your own journeys and have your own needs. Trust Him.

IT'S WISE TO LISTEN TO YOUR BODY

When it comes to nutrition, movement, and all things physical health related, God's already given us our best teacher—our bodies! In large part, we're listening to His wise guidance when we listen to our bodies. Track with me here: God created the earth and everything in it, including our bodies, and called it all good (Genesis 1:31). Then Paul reminded us in the New Testament that even after the fall of humankind everything that God created is still good (1 Timothy 4:4). Therefore, our bodies are good and the mechanisms that God's placed within our bodies to keep us healthy are also good.

Let's dive a little deeper. From a scientific standpoint, everything about this marvelous creation called the human body is designed to keep us healthy. This effort by the body's systems to maintain health at all costs is known as homeostasis. These systems regulate hunger, fullness, cravings, pain, stress, and fatigue. For the most part, what happens in the body goes unnoticed by our conscious minds. For instance, as you read this you likely aren't aware of your kidney filtering out sodium, potassium, and water, and I doubt you can detect your liver as it breaks down your old red blood cells or take notice as your bone marrow produces more in a process called erythropoiesis. Yet, all of it is taking place so you can live at your highest capacity. God knew we'd have more enjoyable and important things to occupy our mind with here on earth, so He designed our bodies to function largely on their own. However, there are bodily functions that require our compliance and when the time is right, the body sees fit to notify us through cleverly designed signals.

We receive messages about when it's time to go the bathroom, how urgent it is, and whether we're dealing with a number one or number two. Our bodies let us know when a cold is coming on and we need to rest. We hear from our stomach when we ate a bad batch of chicken salad. If you're a woman, you might know when you're about to start your period by certain changes in your mood, digestion, overall energy levels, etc. When it's time to sleep, our bodies let us know. Similarly, when we're in the mood for making babies, our bodies also let us know!

None of these signals should produce shame or guilt. Each one helps us to stay alive, nourished, rested, and healthy. Our body tells us when we're hungry and what we're hungry for and when we're full. The issue is not that we can't trust our bodies' signals; we know they're for our good because they were created in God's good design. The issue is that we have ignored our bodies pleas and respond only when they shout. We've believed ourselves to be smarter than God and His design, and so we've sought to "control" our bodies' cues for food and rest by ignoring them. So, those cues become quiet and easier to ignore, but our bodies find ways to compensate for our lack of compliance. Whether it means a loss of a period, an injury, an achy back, or constant fatigue—whatever our body must to do to keep us healthy, it will, even if it has to happen without our help. Of course, the body would prefer we listen and respond by giving it what it needs, whether that's sleep, food, movement, or drink. Further, when we become an active listener to the signals given to us by God for our good, we find that our body is our ally, not our enemy.

I can hear some of you now, "What about when I crave food when I'm not hungry or desire to have sex with someone who isn't my spouse? How can you say that's good? What about gluttony and lust, aren't those from the body?" I'd argue that both of those desires and sins are related to our hearts, and not just our bodies. Our bodies do not signal us to cheat on our spouse or overeat. Our beliefs, thoughts, and emotions attempt to override our body signals in order to get what they want. For example, let's say you decide to have dessert with dinner and eat until you are physically full and satisfied, however you're still holding on to the belief that dessert is bad, or that you can only have it every once in a while. Because you believe this way, your mind urges you to have as much of the dessert as you can right now. Your mind races with thoughts like, I already ate some, so why not have more? And who knows when I'll get another chance. You overeat. Was that your body telling you to overeat or your shame focused belief system? Your beliefs.

The same goes with lust. Maybe you don't feel loved by your spouse or you believe God is angry with you. Maybe you've experienced sexual abuse and are living in shame for it. You may be searching for love and validation from all the wrong places, and one of those places just happens to be from members of the opposite sex. Sure, you may be attracted to someone, but with your heart in the right place it's easier to shake this off. However, if you're desperate for affection, and you allow yourself to daydream about that person until you've convinced yourself that you want to have sex with them. Again, the desire intensified because of a misunderstanding of God's love, due to a false belief, not because of your body's wrong impulses..

Okay, so we've established that we can trust the physical cues our body sends, but what does that look like in a world full of super-sized portions, convenience foods, and paradoxically, an unending stream of fad diets? For many of us, we're so confused on what and how much to eat that we've completely forgotten what hunger and fullness feels like. We've lost sight of the days when we could eat whatever we wanted, when we simply had to tell somebody we were hungry, choose what food on our plate we liked, and eat it until we got full. Every one of us was born eating this way, in response to our internal signals. But once food rules entered in we lost touch with this way of eating, or maybe we were convinced by society that it was wrong.

Food rules can be anything from "clean your plate," to no carbs before bed, to kale is good and pizza is bad. Every one of these externally imposed food rules brings us further and further away from eating based on our body's cues. But there is good news, we can get that inner intuitive eater back! It takes practice. We have to become aware and attuned to our body again. The first way in which we do this is by rediscovering our natural hunger and fullness rhythms and eating accordingly.

Eat when you're hungry, preferably when you're first hungry, and stop when you are full and satisfied. It sounds so simple. But years of dieting and ignoring our bodies make it complicated. So let's start with the average person, let's call him Joe. Joe has a normal relationship with food, he eats all foods, and listens to his hunger and fullness cues. He's never dieted and has maintained a steady weight for his adult life.

Joe is hungry within 1-2 hours of waking up and every 3-5 hours throughout the day, depending on the day and the food he eats at the previous meal. Sometimes if he doesn't eat enough, if he's been active, or for some other reason his metabolism speeds up, he's hungry sooner than 3 hours, that's okay, he eats then too. His body likes his regular routine because it helps him maintain an even blood sugar level, which allows him to have a steady stream of energy and remain mentally sharp throughout the day. In the evening, Joe doesn't feel overly famished and eats a bedtime snack if he feels like it. He goes to bed and sleeps throughout the night, not waking in the middle of the night famished because he already ate enough during the day. Joe is a normal eater. Well, he's what a normal eater would be if we didn't live in a diet-obsessed culture where eating normally is abnormal.

We can learn something from Joe. The average human likes routine, and for the most part, that routine involves eating regularly throughout the day, every 3-5 hours (and sometimes before). If you're new to this whole eating when hungry thing, here's a good place to start. Try incorporating a meal or snack within 1-2 hours of waking and then every 3-5 hours (or before) throughout the day. If you typically skip meals, set an alarm at the 3-hour mark to check in with yourself. Are you hungry yet? Is there food around? If you aren't hungry yet, try again in a half hour. Do this until you're hungry, but don't go past the 5 hours.

Eventually, eating in this way will sensitize you to your body's early cries for food. These hunger cues look different for everyone, but here are a few examples of how they might show up. You may notice that you're suddenly distracted from work or you're thinking about food. This is early hunger. Or, you might feel gurgling in your stomach or notice your mouth watering. This too is early hunger. It's a sign that you need to be on the lookout for food, so that you can eat within 15-30 minutes. Later stages of hunger result in uncomfortable stomach pangs, fatigue, headaches, and even nausea. These are signs that you've waited a too long to eat.

If we ignore hunger signals for too long our body will stop sending them, assuming it's a waste of energy to let you know it's hungry; there's obviously a shortage of food, or else you wouldn't be ignoring its pleas so stubbornly. Eating at the first sign of hunger is associated with better blood sugar control, something everyone can benefit from. In contrast, ignoring hunger, or masking it with more and more caffeine, results in increased stress hormone release, poor blood sugar control, and muscle break down. For these reasons, it's important to become aware of and responsive to hunger signs. By following a regular rhythm of eating for a few weeks, you aren't committing to a lifelong meal schedule but rather retraining your mind to hear from your body. You're setting yourself up for more long-term freedom and confidence with eating.

Now you know how to recognize hunger, but what about fullness? How do you stop eating when full? The first and most important step is making peace with food. When we reject the cultural ideal of good and bad foods and hold on to the truth of the Word of God that all foods are to be enjoyed with thanksgiving, then we free ourselves up to finally stop eating when full. How does this work? I'm glad you asked. It works by eradicating the deprivation or scarcity mindset we have with food. When we know that we can eat a food anytime we want, it becomes less appealing to eat past fullness. And even when we eat highly palatable foods, like ice cream, we may *want* to eat more once we're full, but we now understand that it's okay to stop, knowing that if we choose to, we can always eat more at the next meal.

On the opposite end of the spectrum, if we're worried about feeling full for fear of overeating, we can take comfort in the fact that our bodies are designed to be so much smarter than calories in/calories out, or any other man-made food rule. Eating enough food at meal time to satisfy our bodies for at least 2-3 hours afterwards is not overeating, it's giving ourselves what we need. No matter how uncomfortable this may feel in the beginning, it's God's design and we can trust it. So, what *does* normal fullness feel like? In my opinion, this one is more nuanced than hunger. Fullness feels different for everyone, especially for those of us who have been under eating throughout the day. If you've been restricting food for any amount of time, fullness may feel like bloating and gas and discomfort at first, but as your body adjusts, things will make a turn for the better. For the majority of people, fullness results in food no longer tasting as good as it did with your first few bites, it results in your belly feeling satisfied. In the earlier stages of fullness, you will likely feel that you could eat a little more and still feel good. At later stages, it will feel like there is no more room in your stomach, and at the fullest stages, it may feel like you are spitting food back up and you need a BIG nap. Your lifestyle and your comfort level determine what level you get to. For those who like to go longer periods between eating, you may need to feel fairly full to get through 5 hours with no additional food. For those who like eating every 2-3 hours, you may only eat to the point of just being satisfied. The interval at which you like to eat and the severity of your hunger when it comes meal or snack time determine how full you need to feel after eating. So, experiment and find what works best for you. That's the beauty of this way of fueling your body, it's based on you and your needs, not anybody else's.

Remember listening to your body in this way is akin to listening to God's direction. He has designed your physical body with great wonder so you might live a healthy, abundant life as you glorify Him. When it gets tough to trust your body, remember who made it. Keep renewing your mind with this truth, and the truth that God has given you freedom to eat all foods. The lies of the enemy, shame and condemnation, will try to creep back in to steal freedom. We have to train ourselves to hear the voice of wisdom in all things, including food and exercise. This is how we move further into freedom, not by following more rules. For this reason, I won't talk about specific food and nutrition recommendations until the end of the book. I've found that that sort of information is only helpful when we have a full realization of grace and a deeper knowledge of Christ. Then we'll know His voice and be able to listen and learn as He teaches us all things.

WHOSE VOICE ARE YOU HEARING

If we're to listen to the voice of wisdom put inside us by the Holy Spirit, we need to be able to recognize and discern it from the other voices ringing in our ears. For instance, many of us are listening to the voice of our own shame or the voice of the accuser whispering to us about our guilt. There is the voice of our parents and friends and acquaintances who mean well (or maybe don't), but cause fear or self-doubt to well up within us. There is the voice of rebellion that is clawing to act out against every self-imposed rule and person who wronged us. Then there is the voice of the Holy Spirit, who continually speaks truth, encouragement, grace, and instruction to us. This is the voice we have to tune our ears to hear. When it comes to matters of nutrition, listening for His voice is not unlike any other area of life. Once we weed out the voices we know are false, the ones rooted in fear, hate, rebellion, shame, and condemnation, we can hear the truth of what He's saying.

Sometimes our own education and opinions get in the way of hearing from the Holy Spirit. For instance, I'm a dietitian. I study nutrition for a living. Hopefully by this point in the book, you know that about me. But what you might not realize is that all my nutrition training can be a hindrance to normal eating. It's so easy for nutrition knowledge— which, by the way, is constantly changing with new scientific discoveries—to get in the way of making non-judgmental food decisions. I've had to discern which voices and what nutrition information is helpful and what is not helpful. But through the knowledge of the gospel of grace, I've discovered a few tell-tale signs whether what I'm hearing is trustworthy or suspect.

Trustworthy food thoughts sound like this:

They are guiding in nature and not rooted in fear.

For example, a food thought rooted in fear would sound more like this, "I know I need to eat something before my workout, but all I have is this high sugar cereal, sugar is bad and may cause me to become unhealthy. Also, sugar might make me fat. I better just not eat and go workout anyway."

A trustworthy food thought might say, "I'm about to go workout. I need to eat a snack with some carbs, even though I'm not super hungry, that way I'll have energy for my workout."

See how the second example was more helpful in nature, driving you to take care of yourself and the first was rooted in a fear of becoming unhealthy and gaining weight? The second example resulted in fueling your body for a workout. In contrast, the first resulted in failing to nourish your body.

Helpful food thoughts are emotionally neutral and not shaming.

Shaming Thought: There is nothing "good" here. I'll just have pizza. I'm already blowing it anyway. Why not have 5 more pieces? Forget the salad. I am never going to get this clean eating right.

Neutral thought: There's a choice between supreme pizza and salad at this party. I'll get the pizza because it will satisfy me and provide me with energy. I'll also add some salad, because it'll give me some fiber, vitamins, and minerals, plus I like this salad.

Shaming thoughts usually contain an "I am" or "I am not" statement. They usually result in us checking out from the eating experience, either with overeating or anxious thoughts of restricting and compensating. Emotionally neutral thoughts operate in the concept of balance and moderation. They describe food for its positive attributes and don't get stuck in all-or-nothingness land.

Helpful food thoughts are rooted in self-care and not punishment and restriction.

Punishing thought: I ate a snack an hour ago and now I'm hungry again. Ugh, I have no self-control. I'm not giving into this craving. I need to go exercise to get my brain off of food. Alternatively: I can't believe I've eaten two meals in two hours. I'm not eating for the rest of the day to make up for this.

Self-care thought: It's only been an hour since my last snack, but I feel a little hungry, low on energy, and thirsty. I'm going to honor that and make a meal with what's on hand and drink some water.

Punishing thoughts will push you to restrict, over exercise, purge, diet, or worse. These are not helpful, and often result in feeling more and more out of control with food. On the other hand, caring for yourself means fueling your body when it's hungry. It means resting, drinking water, and moving in an enjoyable manner.

Trustworthy food thoughts set you up to enjoy food and relationships and aren't rooted in comparison.

Comparison thought: I'd like some ice cream with dinner; I shouldn't have any though. I'm tired of being the fat one in our family. I'm going to eat like my sister, she's small and everyone likes her. I'll just get the same salad she's ordering (Later that evening after eating, this person is still craving ice cream. Eventually after eating all the "good" foods she can get her hands on and failing to satisfy her craving, she eats the ice cream anyways).

Enjoying food thought: I'm really craving some ice cream with dinner tonight. I'm going to get my favorite flavor so I can enjoy it more (Savors ice cream and is able to stop when full).

When we compare our food, our bodies, our calling, our stage of life, or our walk with God to anyone else's, it steals our peace and points us to our inadequacies. We end up so focused on our shortcomings that we fail to nurture our unique strengths, and we cease to run our own race. Conversely, when we seek to enjoy food mindfully with friends and family it sets us up for satisfaction and connection. Together with nourishment, these are the quintessential functions of food.

133

I don't share all of these examples to discourage you by pointing out your harmful thought patterns. Rather, I share to encourage you that God is not condemning you. We are condemning ourselves and so is the enemy. When we hear those lies circulating in our thoughts, we can respond with the truth. We can replace those thoughts with what God says. And He says that you are righteous, redeemed, fully known, and fully loved. He says that food is good, that it's to be enjoyed, and that nothing can separate you from His grace. He says you are free from the power of those untrue thoughts. If you have one million harmful thought patterns, He has the power to overcome them all. And He'll always be there, reminding you of the truth. It just takes us believing what He says.

REFLECTION QUESTIONS

1. How does this chapter change your view of self-control? Have you been attempting to use this gift outside of God's definition? How so?

2. Have you believed that your body couldn't be trusted in the past? What heart issues have you been blaming on your physical body? How does realizing that it was designed for your good change how you treat it and listen to it?

3. Do you eat on a normal rhythm or are you out of touch with hunger and fullness? Do you struggle with a fear of fullness? How can you trust God in this area? What steps can you take?

4. What common thoughts do you have about food that you now realize aren't trustworthy? What does God's word actually say about those thoughts?

Chapter 10

THE ART OF BEING A PRESENT EATER

For thus said the Lord God, the Holy One of Israel, "In returning and rest, you shall be saved; in quietness and in trust shall be your strength."

ISAIAH 30:15 ESV

A CRISIS OF BUSY

Have you ever woken up in the middle of the night haunted by all that you have to accomplish the next day? You haven't even set your feet on the ground, but you're doing a mental run through of all ten of your engagements, the fifteen errands you need to run, and the eighty-seven emails, phone calls, and text messages you have to send out. Oh, and in the midst of this, you remember your priorities, making a mental note to ALSO be more loving towards your husband and to try to squeeze in a quiet time or a 10 second prayer. You genuinely desire to love people and spend time with God, but your schedule just seems to get in the way, pretty much every day.

If this sounds like you, you aren't alone. Most of us live in a crisis of busyness. We're juggling so many dreams, good intentions, and relationships, striving to make everything come to pass on our own, right now. We barely have time for the things that matter most to us, let alone bodily necessities like eating, drinking, sleep, and movement. And who suffers as a result? We do, and our relationship with God and with those closest to us: our spouses, families, and dear friends. Busy is truly a four-letter word. If the enemy can't shame us into inaction in God's kingdom, he'll distract us with 1,000 different "things." This crisis is one that affects every area of our lives and our walk with Christ, not just our physical health. When we're too busy to spend time with God, we may miss hearing His voice. We may miss receiving what we need in prayer. We put off the renewal of our mind with His word, because our twisted priorities are pushing us to keep going at break-neck pace.

And what does God have to say about it? He calls us to break from our busyness, he asks us to return and rest in Him. God reminds us that our strength is not in doing more, but in having a quiet soul and in trusting Him (Isaiah 30:15). In order to do this, we have to stop running in our own strength, and we have to listen long enough to hear God's voice.

Maybe it's not that you're running to something, but that you're running away from something and "doing" more, and more is the only way you can see to get out of your pain. But what if God is calling you to come back to Him, to rest in His plan, and to let Him be your deliverer and your strength? Sometimes, when I don't feel well equipped for what God's calling me to, I find myself taking more and more on, trying to get away from it. Honestly, motherhood can be one of these things. When I feel like I'm failing or I don't know how to be a good mom or when I feel like I have no control over my kid's life, instead of stopping and asking God for help, I run. I run to start new work projects, to do chores, to self-help parenting books and techniques. In the past, I would run to a new workout routine or diet plan, but the aching never gets better when I run, the inadequacies only feel worse.

It's only when I give my plans to God, trust Him with my children, and ask for His help that I'm able to pause, hear his voice, and gain the strength that I need. And it's in these moments that I'm able to fully soak up the joy of being a mom.

The prophet Elijah was a runner too. In 1 Kings 19 Elijah found himself literally running away from God's plan, only it was for fear of losing his life and the knowledge of his own inadequacies. When he had run far away, Elijah became so dejected that he asked God to end his life altogether and went to sleep. When he woke and realized to his dismay that he was still alive, God instructed Elijah to stand on the mountain and wait for him.

While Elijah was standing there, the Bible says that there was a strong wind, but the Lord wasn't in it. Next there was an earthquake, but the Lord also was not in it. Again, there was a fire, but the Lord wasn't in the fire. Finally, there was a still small voice, a low whisper, and God was there speaking to Elijah. And what did God tell Elijah to do? He told him to go back where he came from, to the place where God originally called him.

You see, Elijah needed to rest in God's plan. But because he became anxious and fearful, he started to take matters into his own hands. Yet God followed him and put him back on the right path, reminding Elijah that He would be with him and telling Elijah of a group of 7,000 Israelites who needed him.

Will we stop running, complaining, and striving enough to hear God's still voice? And when He calls us to return to him, to do what he's called us to and nothing more, will we listen? Will we rest in His plan, knowing that He has given us people to love and things to do on this earth?

In our busyness, in our anxiety, and in our fear, God reminds us:

Be still and know that I am God;
I will be exalted among the nations,
I will be exalted in the earth.
Psalm 46:10 NIV

In other words, God's plan will triumph. As believers, this should give us hope because God's plan is much better than ours. And His yoke is much easier than the one we attempt to carry ourselves (Matthew 11:28-30). We don't have to keep doing ALL the things in an attempt to control our situation, nor do we need to continue running from the hard stuff. We can slow down, knowing that God alone is our strength and our deliverer. He will fight our battles for us; he's got a plan.

LITERAL STRENGTH IN QUIETNESS

From a physical perspective, being still, present, mindful, quiet, or whatever other word you want to use for not-a-crazy-busy-anxious-mess, quite literally improves our strength and our health, as Isaiah 30:15 suggests. First, being in a relaxed state allows your parasympathetic nervous system, the one responsible for rest, digestion, and reproduction, to take over for a time. When you're in this state, your body can begin to mend, recover, and do things like digest and absorb food, build muscle, regulate hormones, and conceive and carry babies. The stress hormone, cortisol, decreases, a positive consequence if your body's been cranking it on overdrive out as a result of chronic stress. Your body has a chance to check its energy stores and tell you whether or not it needs more food, a signal that cortisol suppresses.

In this rested state, you're better able to hear and respond to your body's cues, a phenomenon that we nerds call body attunement. Further, when you allow yourself to sit down and eat without distractions, to really focus on the task at hand, you'll likely experience more satisfaction from eating, leaving you fuller for longer and eliminating mindless overeating.

If there are areas of your life causing you stress, taking time to rest can help you find an appropriate way to address the stressor. Oftentimes, emotional eating in response to unresolved issues stops. Digestive problems improve. You realize you CAN eat grains when you aren't super stressed out. Better yet, as you slow down to enjoy meal time with your loved ones, you learn about what's going on in their lives, and you're able to offer some encouragement. These are just a few of the food specific benefits of slowing down, of being present, and not focusing on the one million other activities you have to do. But how do we get here? What does it actually look like to be a present eater?

BEING, BREATHING, EATING & SMILING

Being a present eater is not difficult, it's eliminating the heart's need to be busy that is hard work. It's letting go of our idols and remembering the only one that satisfies is Jesus. As we do this, we free up time, energy, and mental space for being present. When we trust God with our treasure, our time, and resources, he changes our heart towards Him. When we ask, He often makes it clear where we need make room for him or let someone else take over a task. As we reshuffle our daily lives, and reform a routine, it's important to leave space for margin. Margin allows for the unexpected, it gives space for God to move and work in your every day. But even more, it gives room for you to rest, and just be present with Him.

Being a present eater is no different; we have to give ourselves enough time, or margin, to eat. This may mean getting up earlier to sit down to breakfast. It could look like blocking out 15 to 30 minutes on your work schedule for lunch each day. Creating time to be a present eater and to enjoy family meals might mean saying no to five different evening extracurriculars for your kids. Making time to enjoy meals, or even just one meal, will look different depending on your life. It doesn't need to be perfect or elaborate, but it does need to happen. God designed meal time to be a time of community, rest, thanksgiving, and enjoyment. It's one way that He gets us to stop and take a break from all our striving, to appreciate all that He's given us.

Now that you've carved out some time just for eating, let's talk about eliminating attunement blockers. An attunement blocker is anything that prevents you from hearing from your body, and in this case, anything that stops you from being present during the eating experience. For most of us, these come in the form of distractions, particularly the electronic variety. I know just how hard it is to put away the phone for 5 minutes, to say no to Netflix during supper, to stop working or reading to focus on a meal. I'm guilty of all of it. And you know what, I hate it. Every time I eat in front of the TV or scroll through social media during lunch I feel unsatisfied by my meal.

What happens is our brains are only good at concentrating on one thing at a time (no, multitasking isn't a superpower, it's a symptom of our crazy lives). If we're looking at our phone, reading a book, or watching TV while we eat, our brain isn't fully processing the way the food tastes. We aren't aware of our stomach signaling that we're full, so we just plow through until we hear the clink of our fork on an empty plate. Besides that, if it's one of those days where we're particularly stressed or under fueled and we reach for the potato chips, the same ones we feel like we're "addicted" to, numbing out with TV until we've eaten way too much only confirms our false suspicion and leads us to lose trust in ourselves around food.

Eliminating distractions and allowing ourselves to focus on enjoying our food and good conversation (if it's available) helps us get in touch with our hunger and fullness cues, but also with what food tastes good and satisfies us. Present eaters leave the dinner table feeling much more satisfied, sometimes from less food, than checked-out eaters do after cleaning their plate. Besides this, eliminating the noise and distraction of electronics or other attunement blockers has the ability to reduce our stress levels, which in turn sets us up for healthy digestion and reduced anxiety around food. Another way to do this, and one the Bible encourages is to give thanks for our food.

When we give thanks before we eat, and ask God to bless our food, we're reminding ourselves that He is our ultimate provider and sustainer. He gives health and He is able to make the food that He's provided us with work in our bodies for good. Being grateful at meal time also helps us to relax and activate our parasympathetic (rest and digest) nervous system. This helps those of us with anxiety about eating stay calm and reduce physical symptoms like bloating and nausea. For this same reason, I often ask clients with gastrointestinal difficulties to take three deep belly breaths before eating. Deep breathing also activates the parasympathetic nervous system, allowing the body to digest food more easily.

You can put these principles into practice at home. Some families have made a habit of going around and having each person talk about their day and share something they're thankful for. One of my single clients finds it helpful to write down three things she's grateful for before she eats breakfast and dinner. If you feel up to it, the act of singing aloud may activate what's called the valgus nerve, which is a part of the parasympathetic nervous system responsible for connecting your brain and gut, putting you into rest and digest mode.[1] Gargling water also accomplishes this.

Regardless of how you choose to do it, once you're in a relaxed state and your body is prepared to eat and digest, you can move on to the next step: mindfully enjoying your food—assuming of course, it's not burnt to a crisp, like the bacon I made last night.

MINDFUL EATING UNCOMPLICATED

So, before any of you get all crazy on me and tell me that mindfulness is new age, woo-woo, or the spawn of Satan, let me define it. Mindfulness is simply paying attention to the present moment, on purpose, without judgement. Does that sound so terrible? Doesn't Jesus himself instruct us not to worry about the future, but to stay focused on today? (Matthew 6:25–34) Paul writes in 1 Corinthians 4:3 that he doesn't even judge himself, so that his conscience can be clear, but instead instructs us not to judge anything before the appointed time when the Lord comes and will bring to light everything. Mindfulness is doing just that. It's focusing on the present moment, on what God's put into our hand right now and leaving out the self-condemnation.

Many confuse the meditation discipline of "clearing the mind of all thoughts" with mindfulness. But we know, as Christians, that when we meditate we FILL our minds with God's truth, even if that means focusing on one word, one verse, or one aspect of His character. When it comes to eating we can utilize both mindfulness and Christian meditation to improve how we relate to food. Mindful eating helps us connect to our food and enjoy it without judging it, or ourselves, for eating it. Christian meditation helps bring our thoughts back to the truth of God's word when our mind wants to stray to anxious, shame-filled thoughts about food. Here's how this plays out.

Imagine sitting down to a distraction free lunch at your desk. You've turned your computer off and put your phone in your bag. You have five to ten minutes to enjoy the homemade chicken salad sandwich, peaches, and dessert you brought from home. After taking three deep breaths to let go of any extra tension and saying a prayer to thank God for His provision of food, you pick up your sandwich first. Looking at it, you see that it's a little smashed from sitting in your lunch box all day, but the bright orange peach beside it makes you excited to dig in. You notice the pleasing smell of the bread as you bring the sandwich closer to your face. The first bite is the best, the flavor combo of mayo, apple, and curry in your chicken salad is your favorite. It reminds you of your mom, it's her recipe after all.

As you continue chewing you're aware of the crunch of the apples and the smooth texture of the bread. Next comes the swallow, you can feel the food as it disappears down your throat for a brief moment and then it's gone. You go for the next bite, continuing in this way until you have a thought pop into your head about work and what you have to accomplish during the next half of the day. You consciously draw your attention back to the present, reminding yourself you have plenty of time to think about work later. As you continue to eat, you notice that the sandwich no longer tastes super good, it's just neutral. You decide to go for your peach. The first bite of the peach is like the first bite of the sandwich, full of flavor and excitement. You finish the peach, enjoying every last bite. The sandwich still doesn't seem appealing, but you could still eat a little something more.

You look longingly to the cookies you packed. Immediately a voice of fear and shame enters your head. "You can't eat that cookie, it's processed and it'll probably make you sick and gain weight." But then a beautiful thing happens, because you've been filling your mind with the truth of the gospel, you have a response for that thought prepared. The Holy Spirit brings to mind 1 Timothy 4:4 and you remind yourself. "All foods are made clean by the word of God and prayer. These cookies are given to me for enjoyment and energy and God will use them in my body for good." You proceed to eat one cookie, enjoying the rich flavor. You finish the first cookie and realize you're feeling pretty full. Wrapping up the rest of your sandwich and the remaining cookie, you put them back in your lunch box in case you're hungry again later. You feel completely satisfied and ready to return to work.

In this scenario, we utilized mindful eating and scripture meditation, or mantras, to help us stay at peace and discover satisfaction in eating. Allowing yourself to notice the sight, smell, texture, and taste of your food, without judgement, makes it easier to hear what foods your body is hungry for and to detect fullness. Using all of your senses in the eating experience promotes a higher level of satisfaction and decreases the chances that you'll be raiding the vending machine for something thirty minutes after lunch. The even more beautiful part of this example was the use of scripture as a short meditation, or mantra, to replace negative food thoughts. This is Romans 12:2 in action, the renewing of our minds and transformation of our lives. But being able to do this requires that we be present to our thoughts and self-aware enough to recognize those mindsets which lead us down dark paths and back into bondage to food.

Mindful eating is not another all or nothing food rule. No one eats mindfully every meal. No, mindful eating is simply a tool you can use to help tune into your body. It's one way to get quiet in the midst of our daily routine. As we practice mindful eating, we'll be able to discern what varying degrees of fullness and satisfaction feel like, unlock a new level of appreciation for different foods and different flavors, and be able to enjoy food more as God intended—without judgement, without guilt, and full of thanksgiving and trust.

REFLECTION QUESTIONS

1. How has the crisis of busyness affected your life? How does it help you? How does it hurt you?

2. Is there anything that God's calling you to do, or not do, in order to spend more time with him and more time on the things that matter?

3. Do you regularly eat meals on the go or with distractions? What's one step you can take to prioritize meal time?

4. Have you practiced mindful eating or Christian meditation? How can you apply these practices to your life? How can they help you?

Chapter 11

FOOD IS A GIFT, ENJOY IT & USE IT

"I perceived that there is nothing better for them than to be joyful and to do good as long as they live; also that everyone should eat and drink and take pleasure in all his toil—this is God's gift to man."

ECCLESIASTES 3:12-13 ESV

EMOTIONS & EATING

Ever had anyone ask you, "Why does healthy food have to taste so bad and unhealthy food taste so good?" Or here's one of my favorites, "If it tastes good, don't eat it." Like what? I hear this stuff almost daily, and honestly, it makes me sad. I know, I know; I used to be that person. I used to believe that being healthy meant eating steamed vegetables, bland chicken, and some boiled brown rice with nothing but a little sea salt or herbs for flavoring.

Sure, I'd oblige by eating flavorless mush for a few days, so would my husband—we were broke college newlyweds at the time, the poor man didn't have much of a choice. Inevitably, I'd find myself somewhere with free pizza and chips—the official college campus meal—and consume copious amounts of what was actually just *okay* tasting food in order to make up for the total lack of satisfaction I was getting from my cooking. It's the same principle as cheat days. Restrict food, either in amount or type, eat meals you don't enjoy, but that fit with your diet plan, and then when Friday night rolls around, go on a bender of all the food you like, but in huge amounts. Once Monday arrives, the terrible bland food returns.

Why do we put ourselves through this? It's not helpful. And if you've read this far, you know that restriction only leads to feeling more and more fearful around food, and oftentimes, to bingeing. Denying yourself the pleasure of enjoying the food you eat is no different. You'll find yourself daydreaming about comfort foods, ice cream, anything that tastes good. And sometimes, in an effort to get a little satisfaction from food, you'll end up eating a whole Mellow Mushroom pizza after you already stuffed yourself full of tilapia, broccoli, and quinoa at dinner. You don't necessarily have to under eat calories or be an "emotional eater"—I'll talk about this misused term later—to end up in front of the TV with an ice cream pint and a spoon. You could simply be craving some enjoyment from food that you haven't allowed yourself to have all day.

God gave us food as a gift to be enjoyed. Yet, our culture, even the Christian culture, tells us that finding pleasure in food is wrong. God invented pleasure. He designed us to crave it and the things that cause it: sex, food, and entertainment. He made all of those things, and when used correctly, they're good things. So how do we use food correctly? It's simple, we enjoy it. We don't make the eating or the not eating of it into our savior.

It's like what Paul wrote to the Corinthians concerning their sexual impurity.

> "I have the right to do anything," you say—but not everything is beneficial. "I have the right to do anything"—but I will not be mastered by anything. 1 Corinthians 6:12 NIV

Yes, you are allowed to diet and cut out certain foods and fast. You are also allowed to overeat and have cheat days and feel sick. But that doesn't make these things good for you. I think we use this verse out of context as an argument for why we should never eat certain "bad" foods. People who have this mindset about food tend to feel out of control around certain foods, so they conclude that they should never eat them. But not eating a food and constantly restricting more and more foods only makes the bondage stronger. And while this verse is about partaking in sexual idolatry, rather than eating food, it's talking about something that is harmful for us and warned against by God. It's not the same with eating food, according to 1 Timothy 4, God does not consider any food bad. Instead, what we're often enslaved to is the act of cutting out more and more food, the high of dieting, the hope of the next clean eating regimen, the opinions of other people, or the praise we get for how our body looks.

Sometimes, we are enslaved to fast food, but not because it's so addicting; because we've given it so much power. We feel that it's a "naughty" food and if anyone knew we regularly ate it they'd disapprove. So, the enemy tells us we need to hide what we eat and how we eat. The allure of the food becomes even greater with secrecy and shame. We are, in effect, enslaved to this food, not because the food itself is so bad, rather because of our own guilt.

We are enslaved to the idolatry of food as our savior and its effects are either under eating and obsession, resulting in shutting down from the rest of the world, or overeating and feeling ashamed, which also results in hiding from the world. The root is the same, an overvaluing of food; the result is the same, isolation. For this reason, consider your freedom with food as a blessing, but remember that submitting again to the idolatry of food is slavery. What's best for you is between you and God, but I urge you to consider carefully your intentions.

There are some of us who try to meet our non-food needs with eating. I've been there. I've used food to distract me from all things I have to do around the house or to calm me down after a crazy day at work. I've shoveled ice cream in the middle of the day, simply to get through the stress of new motherhood. It's okay. It's impossible to separate our emotions from eating. Food brings pleasure. It's a part of family gatherings and cultural traditions. It's used to show love and provide comfort. Just think about breastfeeding. Babies don't nurse just for food, sometimes they nurse simply because they've missed their mom or they got a boo-boo. Nourishment involves emotion.

God designed it that way. But when food is habitually our only coping mechanism, or when we find ourselves eating when we feel uncomfortably full in order to numb out—maybe even to punish ourselves—that's a signal that we have a deep heart need that isn't being satisfied. So, what do we do? We return to the satisfier of our souls. We renew our minds with His truth. We seek Him out to remind us of our worth, to remind us of His love for us, and we ask Him to reveal our true need and to fulfill it. And then we forgive ourselves, because He has already forgiven and forgotten our sins.

Sometimes it feels like this process is an unending cycle: trying to meet a legitimate need with the wrong means and going back to God to ask Him to meet it instead. I think He meets our needs one at a time, instead of all at once, so that we'll continue to seek Him. I've said it before, but our daily need for food is a picture of our daily need for Him. Let's remember that emotions belong with eating. Let's stop judging ourselves for something that's natural, and instead seek to fulfill every need of our soul with Jesus. As we return to Him day after day to meet our needs, we won't have to turn to food, or to restriction. What's left is the simple act of listening to our bodies, eating, and enjoying.

WHY ENJOY FOOD

I'm a hard-headed person. I need to be convinced of almost everything, sometimes even obvious things. But once I understand something and believe it in my heart, it's going to take an act of congress and God to break that conviction. So, for the sake of the stubborn readers out there (like me), the ones who, as children, constantly annoyed their parents with the questions: "Why?" and "How come?" I'm going to lay the groundwork for why we should enjoy food.

From a biblical perspective, it's clear that God gave us food for more than nourishment. Yes, food provides energy and aids in the health of our bodies, but it also serves as a means of communion with God and others. Jesus often ate at the table with sinners to show His love and acceptance. In His time, eating with someone meant that they were akin to family; it was a symbol of your connection with that person. It's one of the reasons why, when Jesus appeared to the disciples and Peter on the shore of the sea after his resurrection, He was cooking them breakfast. Jesus was demonstrating that He was still in bodily form; God had truly raised his body from the dead, and even in His resurrected state He still ate food. But what's more, He was demonstrating that He still loved and accepted His disciple, Peter, even after Peter denied Him three times. And after Jesus ascended into heaven? Acts tells us that the early believers came together and broke bread daily, communing with each other and remembering the finished work Jesus did by giving His blood and body on the cross.

Solomon writes in Ecclesiastes that food was given to man by God to be enjoyed, that eating and drinking and enjoying the fruits of our labor are some of the greatest gifts God gives this side of heaven. But what about the other side of heaven? What will food look like in eternity? I can't say for sure because I haven't been there yet, but I do know that the Bible refers to feasts and trees bearing fruit in heaven (Matthew 8:11, Revelation 22:2). Will we need food in heaven to live? Revelation 7:16 tells us we will never again hunger or thirst, so no, I don't think we'll NEED food. So then, why will we have feasts? Well, if it's anything like earth, feasts are for celebrating, for enjoying life and every good blessing of God's. Just a little more proof that food was made to be enjoyed.

From a scientific perspective, our bodies function best when we eat foods that we enjoy. Research shows that we absorb the nutrients found in food better when the food is appealing and enjoyable. One study [1] looked at two groups of women from two different cultures. They fed each group a traditional meal and looked at the rate of their iron absorption. Then they fed each group the other cultures' traditional food, something they weren't as inclined to enjoy, and looked at the rate of iron absorption again. As anticipated, the women absorbed the most iron from their culture's traditional meal. This is to be expected. Our body gets used to the foods we feed it and can better digest something eaten regularly because it has the right enzymes and bacteria to do the job.

The interesting part of the study is what happened next. The researchers provided each group of women their own traditional meal but blended it up in a smoothie. We would think that breaking down the food before feeding it to the women would enhance absorption, making the nutrients in the food more readily available to the body, however the fact that the food was now an unappealing pile of mush ensured that the women were not enjoying their meal as much. The result? They did not absorb near as much iron as they did when they enjoyed what they ate.

This may partly explain why different cultures can enjoy completely different diets and still be extremely healthy. Our bodies are accustomed to what we eat and enjoy, and they're efficient at utilizing that food for our benefit. Regardless, the conclusion remains, eating foods you enjoy may improve nutrient absorption.

As I alluded to earlier, choosing foods that taste good and allowing yourself to derive pleasure from eating increases the overall satisfaction of your meal. Satisfaction keeps you satiated longer than a meal that simply makes you physically full. Ironically, we're less likely to overeat when we give ourselves permission to eat the ice cream we're craving than when we try to subdue the craving with "health foods."

Once upon a time, I ate a lot of rice cakes. No shame if you like rice cakes. I just didn't. I ate them because they were lower calorie, filler foods. I remember one time having a craving for some toast, but since bread was the root of all evil, I chose to eat a rice cake. And since the rice cake was as bland as bland can be, it needed some jelly. And then the next one needed some almond butter and honey, then the third one needed more jelly with ricotta, then the fourth one…. You get the point. If I had just eaten the toast with some butter, like I wanted to, then I would have had one or two pieces, maybe 250 calories at most! Instead, I consumed rice cake after rice cake and was completely unhappy with a calorie amount that was at least double what the toast would have been. Moral of the story, just eat the toast (or whatever else you're craving) and enjoy it. It's not bad! It's food. It's carbs, protein, fat, vitamins, minerals, energy, and satisfaction—the most priceless component of all.

HOW TO ENJOY FOOD

For some of us this concept of enjoying food is so foreign and scary we need a road map to navigate. Let's layout some step-by-step directions to get from diet land blandness to food freedom and flavor.

First, make a list of your favorite foods, meals, and restaurants. Do you have a certain type of cuisine you're drawn to? What about staple ingredients? Think back to your childhood. What did you like to eat before diet culture tainted your view of food? Hopefully by this point in the book, you've started to work through your fear of foods and are feeling more open to previously off-limit foods you enjoy. If not, go back to chapter 8, the section on overcoming fear foods and follow the steps to squash those food fears.

Next, keeping your favorite foods in mind, make a list of breakfasts, lunches, dinners, and snacks you can make. Buy what you can and keep it in your house, on your person, and available for you to enjoy. If you feel like eating it, eat it until you're full and satisfied. Take note of how it feels to be content after eating vs searching for more tasty food. One caveat: every time you eat doesn't need to be this glorious satisfying experience. Sometimes you have to eat out of a box, on the run, or at a friend's house. Sometimes you have to eat what you have on hand. That's okay. By allowing yourself to enjoy your favorite foods as much as you can, and when it makes sense, you're signaling to your body that eating boring food is alright part of the time because there will always be another opportunity to eat in another two to four hours, and then again, the next time you feel hungry. There is always a chance to enjoy food more at the next meal with no threat of restriction ahead.

Besides getting to know your favorite foods, keeping them around, and allowing yourself to eat them, you can take it one step further by learning how to prepare tasty food on your own. For those of us who already cook, we have to ask ourselves, is what we're making enjoyable to eat or is it bland and reminiscent of diet food?

Full transparency here, when I first started breaking free from food rules, I realized that the stuff I cooked wasn't all that yummy. I quickly figured out that if I wanted to keep some money in our bank account I was going to have to learn how to make food at home that tasted as good as I remembered and better than going out to eat. There were some very simple swaps I made that immediately improved the flavor of our food:

- I started adding fat to pretty much everything I cooked. I use olive oil, coconut butter, butter, avocado oil, bacon, cheese, cream, you name it. These fats come with a lot of flavor and a little goes a long way! Besides, fats have so many benefits, including better vitamin absorption, hormonal health, immune health, and they keep us full longer.

- I started adding real sweeteners to meals, like sugar *gasp*, honey, and maple syrup. I stopped using artificial sweeteners, because one, if we're honest, they don't taste as good, and two, they don't actually satisfy our sweet tooth like real sugar does.

- I began to look for copycat recipes of my favorite meals and learned by trial and error. The internet is a wonderful place, full of unlimited recipes. I would search new recipes and play around until I found a combination that worked for us. I also learned a lot of flavor pairings and cooking techniques from doing this. For instance, I hardly ever make rice or any other savory grain without broth, the flavor is too good!

- I switch up what I'm making. A lot of us get stuck in a rut with our meals. What was once a flavorful supper becomes a boring and humdrum meal, and once again we find ourselves searching for more food after we've eaten. I go through phases with our meals. During the summer, I love grilling, cold pasta dishes, and veggie pizzas. During the winter it's roast and soups, and all the comfort foods. Instead of sticking to the same meals, I reevaluate and find new things to make.

These are just a few simple ways I've brought more flavor to the food we eat. Another way to ramp up the enjoyment factor at meal time is to change up your eating environment. Maybe that means adding flowers to the table, using your nice dishes, or turning on mood music. It could also mean that you aim for an array of colors on your plate to increase the visual satisfaction of a meal. There are countless ways to make food more appealing, just follow your gut and take into account the preferences of the other members of your family! It's not uncommon to see your kid's relationship with food transform as you make good, tasty food available, and allow them to choose what and how much they eat. But even more, as you become more relaxed and happy around food, it's sure to rub off on them!

A WORD ABOUT TASTE SCIENCE

I can hear some of you now, "What if the food I like is not nutrient rich food? What if I only enjoy fast food, Twinkies, and pop?" Your concern is valid. If you've really made peace with food and you no longer feel guilty for eating any of it, but you still find yourself choosing only foods that are highly palatable, taste science has some insight for you. We are ingrained to like what we already eat. So yes, if for the majority of our lives, or the past few years, we've been eating mainly fast food, cookies, and other super tasty foods, that's what our taste buds are going to ask for and expect. However, as we begin to listen to our body and hear what it's asking for, many of us will realize it's asking for something else, like dare I say, some vegetables or some form of fiber. We have a choice: we can honor this ask and feed our bodies some vegetables, prepared as well as we know how, with some fat and some seasonings or even hidden in a dish like lasagna or soup, or to our body's dismay, we can ignore its pleas and continue eating the only foods we've known. The beauty of our taste buds is, with persistence, they can be changed. Research shows a child may need as many as 8-15 different exposures to a new food to like it.[2] Adults are no different. We need to try new foods several times before our taste buds and our bodies get used to them.

I'm not saying that you can't eat the foods that you enjoy now—fast food, processed food, highly palatable desserts—only that if your body is asking for something different you can change your taste buds to crave those nutrient rich foods you don't normally eat, like fruits, vegetables, whole grains, beans, nuts, seeds, meat, fish, and dairy. And if you're going to try giving your body these things, why not make them taste as good as they can? Go back to those flavor-enhancing tips and have a go! Realize that your personal preference may still be for green beans over broccoli, and that's okay! We all have different levels of sensitivity to bitterness, and other flavors, that aren't going to be altered, no matter how much we expose ourselves to a food. It doesn't mean that you're a bad person or that you have to avoid an entire food group like vegetables. Just move on to something else, add some flavor, and give it a try! Everyone can enjoy food and everyone can learn to cook. It just takes a commitment to keep trying, a willingness to fail, and a desire to meet your body's needs.

REFLECTION QUESTIONS

1. Do you believe that food was meant to be enjoyed? Have you been allowing yourself to enjoy your food? Why or why not?

2. What's one of your most positive food memories? How are emotions positively related to food for you? What deeper need have you tried to meet with eating or restricting foods?

3. What are your favorite foods, cuisines, or childhood meals? How often do you eat these?

4. What are some ways in which you can increase the enjoyment of your food? Are there any foods or food groups you want to try that you don't eat now? How can you prepare these foods to be more enjoyable?

Chapter 12

REDEEMING EXERCISE

"For physical training is of some value, but godliness has value for all things, holding promise for both the present life and the life to come."

1 TIMOTHY 4:8 NIV

I'm an athlete. Or at least I was one. Now I'm what my Harry-Potter-obsessed teammates and I lovingly called a muggle—a non-athlete, a regular joe. But I'm okay with that. Being a competitive swimmer for the majority of my life taught me at least a thousand life lessons, not the least of which included how to dress to hide legs that haven't been shaved in four months (coach's orders), how to discreetly pee in a pool, and how to sleep in study hall without being caught. In all seriousness, I learned a lot, I grew a lot and I loved a lot, all because my parents decided to sign me up for summer swim league at the age of six.

Most of what I know about hard work, perseverance, motivation, and even relationships stem from my swimming days. But If there is one thing that swimming did NOT teach me, it was how to have a normal and healthy relationship with exercise.

Before you make any assumptions, I am not going to talk about how evil sports are or how coaches drive eating disorders and body image worries. Although that certainly does happen, that's not my story. And while another person with a different temperament may have come away from my same experiences with a wonderful appreciation of movement and life balance, that's also not my story. By nature, I'm a people pleaser (recovering), I'm also quietly competitive—thank you, Dad. From the beginning, swimming was fun for me, because I was good at it, and I got attention for it. I liked being the best, and I liked being noticed. We all like these things, especially those of us who hold the coveted role of youngest child. But as always happens, there came a point where I wasn't the best, and the attention I was getting for swimming started dwindling away. So, I did what I thought I should to improve, to regain my identity—I worked harder. Convinced that more mileage, more intense workouts, a "cleaner" diet, and a greater amount of outside training would get me back to where I knew I should be, I poured my everything into training. Eventually though, there was nothing left to give and my body started to shut down.

Now, the very thing I prided myself on—hard work—wasn't even a possibility. I was so fatigued at practices that my endurance sets—something I'd previously been pretty good at—became a running joke among my coaches. What's worse, I started running in addition to the 25+ hours a week I spent on swimming workouts—as if that would be helpful?

At first, the running was a way to "stay in shape" in the off season, and I hoped, a way to increase my endurance.

But then, when I suddenly lost 10 lbs. and started receiving the attention I was no longer getting from swimming for my appearance, something shifted. Working out started to become a means for me to change my body. Why not throw in some dieting while I was at it? Needless to say, that ended in a train wreck. After one spring studying, swimming, running, and eating like a bird I ended up with mono. I spent an entire summer getting by on 5-hour Energy shots and napping every spare minute. It wasn't until a year later, after a terrible swimming season, that my parents insisted on taking me to the doctor. The doctor confirmed what we already knew—I had worked myself into the ground. Not only did my bloodwork show I'd had mono, but I was anemic too.

That was my sophomore year of college. At that point, my desire to be a good swimmer was enough motivation to do what I needed to do. I rested, I spoke with a nutritionist, I ate more, and I moved from the mid-distance group to the sprint group (a.k.a shorter, easier practices). Guess what? It worked. I swam much faster my junior and senior years. But when it was all said and done I had no reason to keep caring for my body so well.

I tried finding motivation in changing my body's appearance, but it was a flop. Working out was this all-or-nothing thing for me. In my mind, you either trained like an athlete, every day, for an hour or more, or it was worthless. Fitness culture didn't help this perspective. I'd read articles making claims that the more exercise you did the better off you were; they forgot to talk about the upper limits of safety and burn out. I'd read more articles claiming that sixty minutes a day was necessary for body changes and, I'd buy into them. Once again, body change and disgust were the motivators, and I'd completely ignore the fact that they were talking about low intensity movement, let alone question whether I needed to change my body at all. I would go on spurts, training for half-marathons, running miles and miles until I ended up with plantar fasciitis or hip flexor injuries. My body was tired and sick of being pushed past its limits for so long. And even though resting was the best thing for me, I'd feel endlessly guilty for not working out. The thought never occurred to me that I could just do some lower intensity movement for a shorter amount of time. Swimming had taught me that you either work really hard and complete an entire workout or you don't do anything at all. I'd always had coaches to give me exercise plans, and the fact that I couldn't follow one on my own made me ashamed.

Somewhere along the line, I learned to love myself for who God says I am. I found my identity in Christ, and I realized that I didn't need to find it in how hard I worked, how fit I was, how fast I was, or what I looked like. I had a child, my priorities changed, my schedule shifted, and God began to open my eyes concerning exercise. He showed me that movement was indeed good and beneficial for my body, and that it could be enjoyed. He helped me see that movement could even be used to bring Him glory, but not in the way I'd previously imagined.

You see, in my mind, God was only glorified through movement when I won something. Picture a Super Bowl champion giving a shout out to God for his victory. But no—God showed me that exercise could be redeemed for His glory, even in the mundane activities performed by people with below average fitness levels. All of this I've learned by trial and error, by observing others make mistakes and get back up, and by the Word of God. You can learn it too—doesn't matter if you've never worked out or you're a workout fanatic—God wants to teach you how to redeem your relationship with exercise and how to use it to glorify Him.

MOVEMENT HAS VALUE

First, we have to understand that exercise or movement has value. While it is not as important as pursuing godliness I think it's important to look at all the wonderful things that this gift of God, called movement, can do for us.

I intentionally use the word movement over exercise. For many people, exercise implies a pre-planned workout routine that must be completed as written. For others, the word exercise conjures up images of pain, injury, and failure. For the majority of us there are subconscious qualifiers for what's considered exercise. These qualifiers might include rules like: must last thirty minutes and must involve sweating, pain, or becoming out of breath. All of these qualifiers only serve to *disqualify* us from enjoying the benefits of movement. If we feel that we can't measure up to the standard of exercise, we're likely to just do nothing, or to feel dejected or ashamed. On the other hand, the term movement is straightforward and flexible; its definition is simply *the act of moving*. Movement is doable and movement is beneficial.

The field of neurofeedback has shown that the act of moving our bodies regularly is a powerful way for the brain to stay adept to what's going on throughout the rest of the body. When the brain or the body's control center is more aware of issues in the body it can make adjustments to correct them. However, when the brain doesn't receive the neurological feedback it needs from the rest of the body, in this case, from a lack of movement, it can't make corrections, so instead the brain responds by increasing pain signals.[1]

Think of a time you've ridden in the car for hours on end. Your back starts to hurt, your neck gets achy, and you feel the constant need to wiggle around. Just sitting here typing I have to regularly stop to stretch out my back and my fingers. The body doesn't like to be still for too long. Those achy pains we have that keep us from wanting to "exercise" may be the reason we need to move in the first place. Movement helps relieve discomfort and may actually promote healing by means of neurological feedback, helping the body to mend itself.[1] Isn't our God awesome? He designed our bodies so well. They have so much potential for health, we only have to listen to them and give them what they need. And one of those needs is movement.

Whether it's stretching, climbing the stairs, gardening, doing housework, walking, running, lifting weights, chasing toddlers, riding bikes, or doing some yoga—regular movement has real benefits. These include decreased risk for cardiovascular disease, diabetes, and some cancers; improved mental health, including a decreased risk of depression; improved judgement and learning skills as you age; and better sleep. Regular movement improves quality of life (possibly by decreasing rates of disease and pain and by improving mental acuity and balance as we age).[2] It also increases your chance of living longer. There is no doubt, regular movement is a good thing. However, just like every other good thing, it can be abused. And when its abused, movement can quickly become harmful to our soul and our body

MOVEMENT AS AN IDOL

Just like food, the enemy will do everything he can to get us to give our worship away to movement. After all, that's what it's all about to him, a competition for our worship, praise, and attention. We were designed to worship God, our creator, the only one worthy of our praise. Out of response to God's love and goodness we were meant to adore Him, to enjoy Him in relationship, and to live our daily lives in thanksgiving as worship to Him. But from the beginning there's been a war waged for our praise and worship. In the days of Abraham and Moses, we worshiped false gods, which were often idols we made of the sun, moon, wind, rain, etc.—natural elements created by the one true God for our good. And while it's less common today to pull out a wooden idol and pray to it as a god, we still tend towards giving our worship—our time, attention, and praise—away to the things of this world instead of the God who created it.

Exercise or movement becomes an idol in our lives when we give it our heart. What does it look like to give your heart away to exercise? Jesus told us that where our treasure is, that's where our heart will be also. So, let's get real practical here: Where do you spend your treasure: which is your money, time, and mental effort? Better yet, where do you put your hope and who or what do you give the credit to for your health, happiness, and fulfillment? If fitness or working out gets your treasure or the glory, it's an idol.

Without a proper view of God and His heart for us, we can easily look at all the benefits of movement and turn it into the thing that we worship. But movement doesn't have our best interest at heart. It doesn't know our every thought and love us anyway. It can't provide fulfillment, grace, acceptance, or even complete health. It will never satisfy, and in the end, it will consume more and more of our time until we're broken, physically, relationally, and spiritually. I've met clients who've given up dream jobs, chosen not to become involved in small groups, or hang out with friends in the worship of movement. And all along, they were dying to have some sort of connection with others, it was the reason they started exercising in the first place—to become more likeable, more admirable. Yet their idol isolated them from ever enjoying the relationships God had for them.

If this sounds like your past, or maybe even your present, rejoice because there is grace for you! God is still pursuing you full force ahead. He has already forgiven your sins and forgotten them. We can go to Him and admit our shortcomings and thank Him for His love and deliverance, despite it all. That is the beautiful God we serve, He is gracious and kind, slow to anger and rich in love (Psalm 145:8).

MOVEMENT AS PUNISHMENT

While some of us haven't made exercise our savior, we may be letting something equally sinister dictate how and why we move our bodies—shame. Shame drives us to do all kinds of things, and as far as I know, none of them are good.

When we let shame remain hidden, we allow it to call the shots. Shame's a terrible boss, it asks us to do things that go against our best interest and the well-being of others. However, when we're under its rule, shame's requests seem reasonable, and even necessary. When it comes to exercise, shame orders us to do one of two things: it convinces us to completely give up on movement or it drives us to abuse exercise as punishment.

Shame tells us that we're too far gone, too unworthy, and too disgusting to enjoy movement. It keeps us from going outside, walking, or enjoying our bodies because it convinces us they're unacceptable to people and to God. What a farce. God does not need your body to look a certain way to use you or to bless you. But He does need you to kick shame in the arse and remind it of your righteousness, the worth you have in Christ, and the calling He's placed on your life.

The other way shame affects our movement habits is by driving us to use exercise as a form of punishment. Shame loves all of our self-inflicted rules y'all, because each time we break them, it's an opportunity for shame to lay down the hammer, point us to our shortcomings, and then show us how we can "punish" that indiscretion. When we break movement and diet rules, shame tells us we need to exercise harder, longer, and more intensely. When we feel like we need to rest, it pushes us forward with shouts of, "You deserve this, you're fat, you're lazy, no one will love you unless you work out." On the surface this may sound more like, "I have to work out to earn food," or "I ate that cake last night and now I need to go on a long run." Underneath, the motivation is still punishment, and the punishment is yet another thing we do to satisfy shame's demands.

If shame or punishment is the motivation for us moving our bodies, we won't be able to move in a way that's healthy. Either we'll neglect moving all together or we'll overdo it and hate it. The answer may sound familiar: kick shame right out of your life. Approach Jesus with an unveiled face, be open, honest and vulnerable with Him. Receive His forgiveness, His peace and His guidance. And if you need to, find a trusted friend, family member, or counselor who you know will respond with the grace of God and do what shame hates: expose it, bring it to the light. When we do this, we set ourselves up to receive every good gift, no strings attached. And these good gifts include a healthy relationship with movement, one that's rooted in pure intentions for self-care, enjoyment, and longevity. Sound good to you? Let's dream about what that looks like a little more.

MOVEMENT AS SELF-CARE

It's time that we take back movement and utilize it as the gift it is. Redeeming movement in my life was a trial and error journey of self-discovery, and one that has been rewarding both mentally and physically. Now, I'm able to look ahead to the days in front of me and set my intentions to move throughout the week. Depending on what's going on, and how I feel physically, a week of planned movement might look different. On a normal week, I might plan to do resistance training two times a week and running two times a week. On a more restful week, like during my period, I might plan to do a restorative yoga practice before bed several times a week and walk up and down the driveway in the morning with my toddler. Sometimes, I get into my day and I decide that I'd rather spend my time working or praying or playing with my kiddo, and that's fine. While regular movement does take intentional thought, it doesn't need to be rigid.

I also don't set unrealistic goals or expectations for my movement practice throughout the week because I know this only sets me up for failure. For me, during my current season of motherhood, movement looks 100% different than my college athlete days. My body takes care of me using the opportunities it gets. My appetite adjusts and my energy levels remain high for the tasks I have at hand. If this sounds like the way you'd like to approach movement, I'd encourage you to go on your own journey, guided by the following steps.

1. Decide how much time you can realistically carve out for movement and how many days per week you'll be able to do an intentional workout. The key here is to start small and set yourself up for success. If you meet your goal, you're reinforcing that you can do this: you can take care of your body without rigidity and shame as motivators. For instance, when I first started exercising with a toddler I set out to complete one fifteen-minute YouTube video three times a week. This seemed doable. I could fit the videos in before my son woke up in the morning or after he went to bed. As I continually did this, I was able to add another day of movement and complete twenty-

minute workout videos. Slowly, but surely, I found my sweet spot with movement.

2. Explore different forms of movement. Find something you enjoy doing. This may take a lot of experimentation, but it's worth it. If you have the time and the finances, try different workout classes, dance lessons, or intramural leagues. If you need to workout at home, try walking outside, different home workout videos, or internet programs. There are a ton of free videos out there and paid subscriptions. You could also purchase hand weights, a yoga mat, or other equipment and make up your own routine. Play around until you find something that works. And when you no longer enjoy it, switch it up! The goal is to continue moving, not to become a fitness robot, repeating the same movements day after day.

3. Remind yourself of why you move your body. Journal about the way movement makes you feel. Commemorate the positive experiences so you can look back on them and find motivation. Sometimes we don't feel like moving our bodies, even when we need to, and we need the extra reminder of why we do it. I'm not talking about pushing through sickness or injuries to exercise or dragging your butt out of bed only three hours after you fell asleep to hit the gym. I mean those

times when we've fallen out of the habit of moving our bodies and we just can't seem to remember what's good about movement, besides the fact that we "should" do it. Shoulds are right behind shame on the list of terrible motivators. But if you have a positive memory of the way healthy movement makes you feel, that memory will serve as a far better cheerleader. Sometimes we dread doing things that are beneficial for us, but when we finally do them, we find ourselves enjoying them and wondering what all the dread was about. This can happen with movement, so let's circumvent it by reminding ourselves of the positives. In order to do this, we have to first find something we enjoy and then listen to our body to find a level of intensity that is equal parts challenging, energizing, and relaxing, depending on what we need. Once we've done this, the only work is in reminding ourselves that this movement is good, helpful, and totally worth it!

MOVEMENT AS WORSHIP

First Timothy 4:8 reminds us that physical training has value. But it also points us to the greater value of godliness, which holds promises for both this life and the life to come. That word godliness or *eusebeia* in the Greek, literally means a sacred awe or respect, a reverence for God.[3] In order to obtain deep respect and reverence for God, it follows that we come to know him more to fully appreciate His character. Taking that into consideration, what would it look like to incorporate godliness into movement? What if we could use movement as a means to worship God and know Him more? That to me, would be the total redemption of movement: taking it from an idol that the devil uses to steal the worship from God and transforming it into a tool we utilize to give praise back to our heavenly Father. This *can* happen. When it does, it's amazing how much more rewarding and refreshing movement becomes.

So how do we do it? How do we use movement to know and revere God more? There are several ways, but the essence of each is the same. Whenever, however, and wherever you decide to be active, use the time to lean in to God, to pray, to thank Him for the gift of movement, and to worship Him. Use the time to listen for His voice, to shut down the screams of the world and the lies of the enemy, and to be still in spirit while moving.

Practically this might look like listening to an audio recording of the Bible while moving, it might mean listening to a podcast or turning on your worship music. It could look like praying as you walk, stretch, or clean the house. Godly movement could mean doing a yoga practice that revolves around God's Word, or meditating on scripture as your breath in and out and move your body. God is moving in the area of fitness. He's raising up influencers who are creating a way for people to know Him more while they exercise. There are things like Holy Yoga and faith centered workout podcasts. Not to mention the advent of audio books and free Bible apps that read scripture aloud. Any time is a good time to know God more, and the opportunities to do this expand each day as God calls His children to use their unique gifts for fitness and for His glory. If this sounds like something you're interested in exploring, don't miss the resources page at the back of this book, where you'll find specific recommendations for podcasts, websites, and apps to help you on this journey.

Redemption is a beautiful thing. God is taking every part of creation, every good gift He designed for us, and bringing it back to its original purpose. He's making everything new, even those things the enemy has tried to use for our demise. He has already won every battle, and in Him we too are conquerors and co-laborers, working alongside Him to bring life into the dead parts of this world. That means we have to move, move in response to His leading, move on behalf of the hurting in this world, and move despite the lies of the enemy. You've been set free to move, but you don't do it on your own, you do it with the king who reigns forever.

REFLECTION QUESTIONS

1. How do you view movement? Is it something you feel like you should do, have to do, or get to do? How has the enemy used exercise to shame you or to steal your worship?

2. What's a realistic movement routine for you? Have you been setting unrealistic expectations or pushing past your body's signals for rest? What forms of movement do you want to try?

3. What rules do you have around movement, right now, that you need to let go of? Examples may include time, intensity, or type of movement.

4. How can you use movement to know God more, to worship him, or to hear from him?

Chapter 13

CONQUERING BODY IMAGE STRUGGLES

"Jesus replied: "'Love the Lord your God with all your heart and with all your soul and with all your mind.' This is the first and greatest commandment. And the second is like it: 'Love your neighbor as yourself.'"

Matthew 22:37-39 NIV

"I praise you because I am fearfully and wonderfully made;
your works are wonderful,
I know that full well."

PSALM 139:14 NIV

Body image. It's one of those things we ignore. We pretend we don't care, because honestly, it's annoying to still feel insecure as a thirty-year-old or a fifty-year-old. It feels stupid, wrong, shallow. But just like every other hidden thing, if we don't bring it to the light we'll never find healing. And the truth is, the majority of us struggle with it. From age six, all the way to age 100, we worry about how we look and how others perceive us. We feel uncomfortable in our bodies.

Sure, some days we feel great and others we feel just okay, but the point is we all think about it at some point.

I remember staring at myself in front of the mirror as a little girl, often dressing up in my mom's clothes and pretending to be a famous singer/songwriter. I guess you could say, I loved myself. And really, I don't know that I thought about my body at all. I was just enjoying the person God made me to be, which just so happened to be a dramatic little girl with a flair for words and a love of the spotlight. At some point in my teenage years I started becoming aware of my body and how it compared to the bodies around me. I noticed that while other girls were maturing and getting attention for it, I was staying pretty much the same. In fact, the only thing that seemed to be growing was my ever-widening swimmer shoulders. I watched my mom and my older sister fuss over their bodies, like most women do, and I took that in. At some point, some teenage twit called my face cute, but said my body was just "okay." My experience isn't so different from most women. In fact, it was probably much easier than many because I was privileged enough to be born into a body that is smaller, taller, and more socially acceptable. I was blessed to escape childhood without physical or verbal abuse from family or loved ones, something that many cannot say.

Our culture communicates in the dialect of bodies. We emphasize certain bodies as good and others as wrong. We talk about them, complain about them, blame them for everything that goes wrong, or in turn, give them glory for all that's going right in our world. Oftentimes our body image struggles aren't an issue of how we look, but a sign of a deeper heart need we're unaware of. Our body becomes the scapegoat for us to ridicule when things aren't working out the way we'd like.

If unmet needs are at the root of our body image struggles, then it follows that changing our body shape will not solve the problem. I've seen the opposite. Someone struggling with anxiety or insecurity may turn to controlling food and manipulating their body shape in an attempt to find peace and identity. When extreme restricting results in losing weight, society responds. We've been trained to give compliments on weight loss and appearance changes. It's what you're supposed to do. But according to who? I'm not sure. The positive attention that a person receives for their appearance only reinforces the idea that our bodies are both the cause and the solution to all our problems. The root problems of anxiety and insecurity are still there, and in an attempt to retain the positive attention there are few limits to how much deeper they may go, fighting to maintain the weight loss and restriction. This can't go on.

We have to get to the root of our bad body image and stop relying on the twisted opinions of the world, the ones that say weight loss and muscle tone are the solution to all ailments. We have to learn to love ourselves for who we really are because ultimately, we will leave this body behind one day and the only thing that will remain is the person God created us to be. Will we choose to love that person now or wait to know her until eternity, drowning her out for our entire stay on earth with all the noise about changing our bodies? If you choose to keep hating on your body, would you change your mind if I told you Jesus, himself commanded us to love ourselves?

WHAT YOU'RE MISSING IN THE GREATEST COMMAND

In Matthew 22:36, the Pharisees ask Jesus what the greatest commandment is. They're trying to trip Him up. Because He's the son of God, He answers perfectly, telling them to love the Lord with all their hearts, minds, and souls and to love their neighbors as themselves. If you've been around church for any amount of time, you've probably heard this before. But what you might not have realized is this: Jesus is commanding us to love ourselves. How can we love our neighbors as ourselves, if we do not first love ourselves? Think about it. You treat people, especially the ones closest to you, the way you treat yourself. If you hold yourself to impossible standards and believe that you can earn God's grace, chances are you have pretty high standards for your loved ones and a hard time seeing past their faults. I know because this was me (and sometimes still is). Jesus gives us the solution. Love God with all your heart, mind, and soul. And the only way we can do that is if we get to know Him. We can't love someone fully without knowing them fully. Jesus understood that knowing God would deepen our love for Him, because He knew first-hand just how gracious and loving God is. The result of knowing God is a thankful heart, one that loves Him back. From this place we begin to see ourselves as God sees us, whole, blameless, fearfully and wonderfully made, called, and set apart. When we see ourselves this way, we start to love ourselves rightly, and from this place of love and confidence we can love other people without threat of losing the worth or acceptance that comes from God.

Is it hard for you to believe that God loves you as you are? Do you hear a million voices reminding you of your faults or the things that have been done to you in your past? Remember that while you may not be able to stop those voices from screaming right now, you can choose whether you believe them and fight back with the truth. You can choose whether you meditate on the lies or actively fill your mind with the knowledge of God. You are loved. Which by definition makes you loveable. Not in the future when you change your body, but now, just like you are.

CONNECTION NOT COMPARISON

The root of body image struggles could be any number of things: insecurity, uncertainty, fear, anxiety, loneliness, trauma, cutting words from a loved one or a schoolmate—but at the bottom of many of these is a deeper root of disconnection. Disconnection from people, disconnection from God, disconnection from ourselves, disconnection from our bodies. When we feel disconnected, or the threat of disconnection, we tend to turn to body bashing. Think about it, have you ever been nervous for a social event where you'll have to meet new people? How many outfits did you try on getting ready for that event? How many times did you pick at yourself in the mirror? This is an example of us being fearful of disconnection. We want to fit in, to be accepted by and connected to the people around us. Or maybe you've experienced real rejection from a loved one or a significant other. Maybe they verbally insulted your body. Or maybe you've experienced physical trauma or sexual abuse, and that's led you to completely disassociate from your body and isolate yourself from relationships. Can you see how that disconnection from your body and other people drives you to hate your body more and more?

This is not an easy issue to talk about, and I don't pretend to understand it completely, or to know what it's like to experience trauma on my body. What I do know is that God understands and He aches for every injustice that has been done to you, big and small. He does not cause these things to happen and He certainly didn't design you or your body for harm. However, He is faithful to take every wrong thing that has happened to you, and every bad situation, and use them for your good. He will use what the enemy intended for evil and redeem it for your benefit and His glory. The journey of healing our body image begins with this process: allowing the Father who loves you to heal your wounds, to show you that you are connected to Him, etched on His heart forever, and then to allow Him to tear down the walls that keep you disconnected from the rest of the world.

Next comes our part, remaining in Him. We must stay rooted in who He says we are and what He's called US to, resisting the urge to find acceptance in people. After all, Paul urges us in Romans 13:8 that we have no obligation to any man, but to love him. You are not called to beat people, to impress them, to please them, or to be like them. We are each unique and comparing ourselves to others around us only serves to make us feel more disconnected from them. It distracts us from what God is calling us to do and causes us to focus on our shortcomings. So instead of comparing ourselves to people, let's connect with them, let's love them as we love ourselves, and build them up as they follow God's calling on their lives, which may or may not look similar to our own.

Practically, this might mean unfollowing accounts on social media that make you feel less than or that tend to lead you into the comparison hole. No, this isn't mean or hateful. People don't know when you unfollow them and, you may find that as you give God your heart and behold more and more of His character that you are no longer tempted to compare yourself to others. At that point you might be able to re-follow that person. The same goes with the company you keep. You've heard it said that you become who you spend your time with. Now, am I saying that you should cut people out of your life completely and tell them it's because they're toxic? Absolutely not. Jesus hung out with the unlovely; He ministered to the toxic people of His time. But He was selective about the people He spent the majority of His time with, His disciples. And even within His disciples, you'll find Him interacting more with a select few. You can love people and spend time with them while also setting boundaries. Only you know what that looks like with the people in your life. Remember that when we do this, we also ought to be surrounding ourselves with believers who will lift us up in Christ. Try replacing the time you might have spent comparing and tearing yourself down with time spent getting to know God through His people.

It's in authentic godly community that we experience being fully known by other human beings and fully accepted. It's the closest we get to experiencing the love of Christ in another person. Even if you don't have that yet, I'd encourage you to remember that God alone will meet your deepest need for connection, and then He will supply people to be a reflection of that, but with Him, you can start now, no need to wait until that little body bashing monster starts singing again.

TRUSTING THE GOD WHO MADE YOUR BODY

As you embark on the journey to love yourself and accept your body, remember that you are not just trusting your physical body to care for you, but the God of the universe, the one who created your body, your heavenly father. It can be difficult to trust a body that's encouraged other people to throw insults at us, or maybe one that's been physically abused. It can feel impossible to trust something that's seemingly caused so much pain, maybe as the result of a chronic illness or injury, but it is not your body that is the problem. It's not your fault either. We like to blame our bodies, ourselves, and even God. He says you are fearfully and wonderfully made, that His work is good. He is not the author of evil or disease. He says He is our healer. If you will trust this, trust Him: He will redeem your relationship with your body, no matter how unlikely it seems.

In the meantime, as you learn to accept, respect, and appreciate your physical body, take action now towards loving it well. I'm talking about practical things like buying clothes that fit you, that you like, and that are comfortable. And yes, this also includes traditional self-care behaviors like taking regular showers, doing your nails, brushing your hair and teeth, moving your body, and sleeping and feeding yourself regularly; we've discussed many of these things in this book.

Hopefully, you're starting to understand just how precious you are to God and just how worth caring for you are. But on those bad days, because they will come, we can send a big message to the enemy of our hearts by continuing to care for our bodies, despite how we feel. And we do it because we get to, because God calls us whole and blessed, not because we should or because we need acceptance from other people. This is the part where I think our rebellious nature serves us, when we use our rebellion to stick it to the man—in this case the accuser, the devil. "Not today, Satan." I find myself saying this Christian pop-culture statement when those anxious body image thoughts begin creeping in and when shame tries to convince me I'm not loved. And my rebellious action is to eat anyway, to rest anyway, to get dressed and do my hair anyway, to go on a walk with my son, or to post that picture. We can find ways to fight the lies of the enemy and hold onto our peace by continuing to care for our bodies. And that's something this strong-willed girl can get behind. What about you?

REFLECTION QUESTIONS

1. Think back to the last time you had a bad body image day or moment. What was going on that day? Was there something else at the root of those negative emotions?

2. How has disconnection or the fear of disconnection driven you to dislike or mistrust your body? How is God calling you to respond to that?

3. Do you have a community or a friend that you'd like to connect deeper with? What's holding you back? Ask God to reveal this and change it!

4. What can you do or say on the days that you feel body shame rising up? How can you use that rebellious nature to defeat the enemy and love yourself well?

Chapter 14

NOURISHMENT BY GRACE & THE SPIRIT

"Yet we don't see ourselves as capable enough to do anything in our own strength, for our true competence flows from God's *empowering presence*. He alone makes us adequate ministers who are focused on an entirely new covenant. Our ministry is not based on the letter of the law but through the *power of the* Spirit. The letter of the law kills, but the Spirit pours out life"

2 CORINTHIANS 3:5-6 TPT

"What's your primary reason for seeking nutrition counseling?" It's a question I ask every one of my new and potential clients. The answers vary every time, but one that I've heard over and over again goes like this: "I'm just confused on what to eat. I want to eat healthy, but I don't want to diet." Or better yet, "I just want to know what to eat." It sounds kind of silly when we think about it.

How is that we, the human race, the most intelligent species on earth, are at a loss for what to eat when seemingly every bug, bird, fish, and beast has no problem figuring this out?

Maybe it's that we're too intelligent, and we overthink everything, including food. Or maybe it's that we're extremely social and prone to base our habits on other people's opinions, as opposed to instinct and personal experience. One thing's for sure, we're confused and it's not for a lack of information. If anything, we have an extreme oversupply of *conflicting* information. Hopefully by this point you've become at least somewhat convinced that there is no one right way to eat, that each of us has unique preferences and needs when it comes to food. Ideally, you understand that listening to your body is a far more effective means of feeding yourself than listening to a diet book, even a well written one, backed by the latest research. As I mentioned before, nutrition research is constantly changing, and if there is one theme it's this: we humans are extremely adaptive creatures who can thrive on all different types of food from lard to lima beans, white rice to coconuts, red meat to tofu. In light of all of this, I am very careful with the nutrition recommendations that I give, working with individuals to help them decide what food patterns work best for them. Together we decide what foods to incorporate and what habits to nurture to improve their overall quality of life.

That being said, there are some basic tenets of healthful nutrition that we can look to. And with all the fad diets, misinformation and over exaggerated nutrition research out there, I do think it's worthwhile to discuss them here.

BUT FIRST...

Please understand, I've chosen to put this chapter at the very end of this book for a reason. If you've skipped the entire book to read it, you're going to be sorely disappointed. Besides that, you will have missed the most important message, the message of grace for eating. Even with the "right" nutrition information, it's nearly impossible to implement nutrition knowledge in a way that is both psychologically and physically nourishing without having a healthy relationship with food first—one that is rooted in truth and grace, and not fear. Only you know if you're in a good place to receive nutrition guidance or if it will become another rule or law to follow, and then to break and feel shame over. Just because you've made it this far in the book doesn't mean you have to be ready for this chapter. Take this journey at your own pace, the pace of grace.

Let's talk about what making health changes with grace and the Spirit's leading looks like. First, it's just like it sounds, Spirit-led, not self-led. God will either put it on your heart to make a change or tell you through His instrument, your body! For me, this has looked like my body repeatedly reminding me that it does not like to go without water for long. This came in the form of headaches and a dry mouth. So, I did the logical thing, I started carrying a water bottle with me and drinking more water when I could. Another simple change I felt led to make had to do with incorporating regular movement. I found myself having difficulty falling asleep at night, adding in some activity relieved this. Finally, I felt God lead me to decrease my caffeine intake after I noticed I was becoming increasingly dependent on it and felt more anxious after drinking it. Here's a perfect example of my nutrition knowledge coming in to play. I knew that caffeine sometimes affected people in this way from my work experience, so it was easier for me to figure out what needed tweaking.

These are just a few personal examples of ways God directed me in habits that were right for ME. You may find you need to make different adjustments. We are each unique. And if you need further help deciding what would work for your lifestyle, I am a huge proponent of getting that help in the form of a non-diet nutrition counselor.

The next component of grace fueled habit change involves focusing on just one or two small changes at a time. God rarely asks us to change everything at once. He knows we can't do this effectively, and better yet, we typically don't need to change, or don't have the means to change, everything about how we're caring for our bodies. From a health behavior perspective, people who make small changes are the most successful in maintaining those habits.

Again, the key is to choose something God is leading you to or your body is clearly asking for. And no, this is not where you convince yourself that your body is asking for a two-week juice cleanse. This is where you listen to your body's craving for carbs and sweets and feed it more carbs. Sure, your body may be asking for more fruits and vegetables, but that doesn't mean it ONLY wants fruits and vegetables. This brings me to my next point: when making changes to your diet, focus on what you can ADD, not what you can take away.

Adding food groups or nutrients that you're lacking is a far more effective strategy for improving your overall diet than cutting away the less nutritious foods.

2 Corinthians 3:5-6 reminds us that we are not capable of doing anything good in our own strength, but instead accomplish God's good plan for our lives through His guidance and empowerment. The same goes with our health habits. We may have all the nutrition knowledge in the world, but if we aren't giving God the control over our lives, if we aren't trusting and listening to God's direction, or if we aren't honoring the needs of the body that He gave us, we'll fall short. You see, if we really believe He is the God who raised Jesus from the dead, if we truly understand that He will also raise our bodies from the dead, then we must realize that He is more than capable of managing our living bodies!

This is not a time to second guess every leading of the Spirit or to examine every craving of your body. If you continue to steep yourself in God's grace, giving all power in your life over to Him, if you keep putting shame and fear in their rightful place, you CAN trust your instincts. You won't have to think hard about the ones that aren't from God. I'm looking at you, three-day long food fast in the midst of eating disorder recovery. Cutting out gluten and dairy, with no signs of food intolerances, I'm looking at you too.

The point is, now that we know the truth and have brought to light the lies, we don't have to question what health decisions are from God and which ones are designed to distract us from Him.

Once we have direction from the Holy Spirit, what's next? Well, we step out in faith and obey Him. And what do we do when we don't see or feel a tangible difference in our health or when we continue to feel anxious about food? We keep going. Faith is not faith if we see the results of our actions right away. Faith is "the assurance of things hoped for, the evidence of things not seen" (Hebrews 11:1). God will lead you into all good things as you follow Him, that includes health.

God definitely wants you to be healthy. However, we have to remember that health is not about a body size. It's about heart posture, psychological well-being, and physical vitality. This is the kind of health God wants for you, a health that doesn't sacrifice any part of your soul. So whatever God calls you to do, do it and have faith that He is using it for your good. You only need enough faith to give the control to Him and get back to living your life without food preoccupation. Remember that we are all in process, and ultimately our life is not about perfection. It's about growing, learning, and loving on the journey.

BACK TO THE BASICS

So where does that leave nutrition education? What's the point if God just leads us to every good thing or if our bodies will tell us what they want? I believe God uses people to speak into our lives and lead us to the answers we need. It's very possible to feel a need to make a change health wise and not have the knowledge to know what to do. That's where health information comes in. If done properly, nutrition education can be empowering, and that's what I hope to do over the next few pages: empower you.

What you will find here: vetted nutrition recommendations that are accepted across the board. What you won't find here: you won't find me talking about outlier research or about ways of eating that have been shown to be helpful for one specific population for a short period of time, but not for everyone. And with good reason, you also won't find me talking about eating for any particular disease state. First, if you're interested in tailored medical nutrition recommendations, I highly suggest working one-on-one with a non-diet dietitian. Second, the general nutrition principles I'm going to discuss are beneficial for most people, which include those with many common chronic diseases. As with everything, you will tweak the amounts and types of food you eat based on your own preferences and your hunger!

Finally, I will not be mentioning the forms of eating that promote the most weight loss, because the truth is we don't know! Most of the studies on weight loss are short term and the ones that check back in, in a year to two years almost always find participants have regained the original weight, and often more. So instead, here are the basics of nutrition: recommendations that help most people.

MODERATION & SATISFACTION

Moderation simply means that you eat portion sizes that are appropriate for your body. This is the principle that we've spent the majority of this book discussing. And as we know, eating the right amount is not a product of counting calories or grams, or measuring out portions. Eating the right amount for your body simply means listening to your cues, eating when hungry, and stopping when comfortably full. It means allowing yourself to eat satisfying foods in amounts that feel good for your body. It means eliminating external food rules that cause you to ignore your hunger and fullness, swinging back and forth between way undereating and way overeating. When you learn to listen to your body, to eat when hungry, and stop when you're full and satisfied, portion sizes become irrelevant. You will eat the amount you need. A little undereating and overeating are nothing to fret over. Your body will adjust your appetite and the energy it uses throughout the day if it has a little extra or a little less food. And so, this tenet of nutrition wisdom goes something like this: eat foods you enjoy and those that make you feel good, mostly when you're hungry; eat them in amounts that your body is asking for, and stop when you're full.

BALANCE

The second biggest piece of nutrition wisdom to observe is balance. In general, our meals and overall diet should contain a balance of the major macronutrients: carbohydrates, fat, and protein, as well as micronutrients like: fiber, vitamins, and minerals. Part of eating a balanced diet is allowing yourself to eat a larger variety of foods. We'll address that in the next section. For those who've struggled with disordered eating, chronic dieting, or restricting, for those who are just beginning to fuel their bodies regularly with all foods, maybe after a long period of following food rules, I suggest a basic pattern for meals and snacks. On top of eating at regular intervals to relearn natural hunger and fullness cues, focus on including each of the following with meals: carbohydrates, fat, protein, fiber, and pleasure. The amount you eat of each is completely individual and based on what you're hungry for. Having a little bit of each of these components ensures a balanced meal and provides the greatest level of satisfaction and fullness between eating times.

CARBOHYDRATES

Carbohydrates include foods made from grains like bread, pasta, rice, cereal, oatmeal, crackers, etc. They include starchy vegetables like potatoes, corn, and peas, along with fruit, dried fruit, and sugar. They are also plentiful in beans and legumes of all varieties. Carbohydrates are our bodies preferred fuel. The brain, muscles and red blood cells thrive off of carbohydrates. This is the one fuel that I see the most fear around, but it may also be the one fuel that has the capability to help you feel more at peace around food. When we go without carbs for too long, it messes with the hormones that signal fullness. As the carbohydrate debt gets bigger and bigger, our bodies drive us to seek out more and more carbs, to become more focused on food, and ultimately to binge on carb rich foods. Eating carbohydrates consistently throughout the day keeps our brains fueled, our bodies energized, and our appetites in check—and that's just the tip of the iceberg. The amount of carbohydrates you need and want will change throughout the day and vary from week to week and season to season, depending on your stress level, your hormonal cycle, your activity level and more. That's normal and okay, and it's important that you honor those needs with a consistent supply of carbohydrates.

FAT

Fat has received a bad rap over the years. It wasn't until recently that popular media and medical professionals started changing their tune about this nutrient. Now, we have the opposite occurring, fat's being touted as THE super food. We went so far to one extreme that now we're compensating by swinging full force to the other extreme. Fat *is* beneficial for our bodies. Besides providing a rich source of energy and cushioning our organs, it helps regulate our hormones, keeps us full between meals, aids in the absorption of fat soluble vitamins A, D, E, and K, coats the nerves in our brain, and aids in fighting inflammation. Fat can be found in full fat dairy like butter, yogurt, and whole milk. It's in oils like olive oil, avocado oil, and sesame oil, as well as avocados, coconuts, and other nuts and seeds, like almonds and flaxseed. Fat is also found in fish, eggs, meat, and poultry. All fats are fair game. We've found that naturally occurring fats found in animal products, plants, and oils are better for our health than processed trans fats (partially hydrogenated oils). However, our body is more than able to handle a little bit of less than ideal fat from time to time. In general, choosing a variety of different fats for cooking with and eating ensures you'll meet your body's needs and avoid nutrient imbalances.

PROTEIN

The third energy providing macronutrient, protein, gets a lot of publicity. Who am I kidding, all of the macronutrients get publicity both good and bad. The reality is that we need all three and none of them are bad, nor are they the panacea for all our ailments. Protein gets a lot of the spotlight because it's a primary component of our muscles and muscles are "so hot right now" (excuse my Zoolander reference). In all seriousness, protein is a pretty important nutrient (just like the others). It helps us build and repair tissue in our bodies, both our own, and those of any babies we're carrying. Protein is an integral part of the enzymes and hormones that are responsible for thousands of metabolic processes in our body. Protein is so important that if we don't eat an adequate supply, our body will start eating its own lean tissue to meet its needs. Protein helps us become full at meal time and stay full between meals—are you seeing a trend here? We get protein from animal foods like eggs, poultry, fish, meat, and dairy. We can also get protein from plant sources like beans, legumes, nuts, seeds, and whole grains. The protein we get from plants is incomplete and less available than the protein from animal foods. So, if we're following a mainly plant based diet, it's important to consume what's called complementary proteins together to make up a complete protein. Complete protein combinations include things like wheat toast and peanut butter or rice and beans. Whether you eat mainly animal protein, or plant protein, is dependent on your preferences and may vary from day-to-day and meal-to-meal. However, those who do not eat much dairy, eggs, or animal protein may consider taking a supplement with vitamin B12, Iron, Zinc, and Calcium to avoid deficiencies.

FIBER

Fiber from fruits, vegetables, whole grains, beans, legumes, nuts, and seeds plays an essential role in our digestive health. It also helps keep us feeling full between meals and provides a rich source of nutrition for the good bacteria populating our guts. Those little guys do good work for our bodies and deserve to be treated well. You can include fiber in your meals and snacks in different ways; it doesn't always have to be in the form of raw fruits and vegetables. And actually, you're free to NOT include fiber in your meals. I certainly don't always eat a perfect fiber source, and there may be days when you want your digestive system to calm down. In such a case, limiting the fiber may be appropriate. But for when you DO want to include fiber, you have choices. You may choose to eat a meal with whole grains, a little protein, and a little fat, and no fruits or veggies. Let's say it's a peanut butter and jelly sandwich with milk. The whole grain bread provides you with carbohydrates and fiber. The peanut butter provides you with fat and a little protein, and the milk provides you with a little bit of all three: carbs, fat, and protein. The jelly gives you some carbohydrates and flavor. That folks, is a balanced meal. Most foods contain several macro and micronutrients. We're just trying to bring in a little bit of everything. It doesn't have to be complicated or stress inducing. There are no numbers to aim for, just food and the energy and satisfaction that comes from eating.

PLEASURE

The last, but necessary, component of a balanced meal (at least in my opinion) is pleasure. We've talked about the importance of enjoying our food and finding pleasure in the eating experience. This pleasure component may look different for you than for me, but in general it comes from any food, nutrient, or spice that provides you with flavor, meets your cravings, and leaves you satisfied. Some common pleasure foods include sweeteners like sugar, jelly, honey, and maple syrup or drinks like iced lattes, Kombucha, or soda pop. Pleasure may mean adding a little extra salt or fat to your food or topping that taco with cheese AND sour cream. It may mean serving up a slice of pie or a brownie with your meal. It could just mean cooking food that you like to eat and enjoying it. Obviously, every eating experience won't be amazing and pleasurable, but if we can aim for pleasure regularly, we'll avoid the feeling of deprivation that often results in extreme, long-term overeating.

At snack time, I suggest clients focus on getting at least two of the three major macronutrients for optimal satiety. After you eat in this manner for a time, you may start to notice little nuances in the way your body prefers to eat. Maybe you like a little less protein in the morning and more meat at night. Maybe you don't feel like you need a lot of fiber in the evenings or you prefer more carbohydrates than fat during lunch.

You do not have to have a "perfect" balance every time you eat (if there even is such a thing). In fact, when we observe how toddlers eat, the perfect intuitive eaters, we see that they eat pretty sporadically, choosing to eat only fruit at one meal and only meat at another, going on kicks of eating mainly crackers, followed by a night of scarfing down tons of broccoli. What we've found is that toddlers get all the nutrients their bodies need over the course of a week.[1] So, while each individual meal doesn't appear balanced, a toddler's cravings naturally drive them to achieve an overall balance over the course of a week. We have this same capability within us, only many of us have gotten out of touch with it. For this reason, we can start with a little structure, aiming to eat regularly, and eat in balance, and once we feel comfortable hearing from our bodies we can take the training wheels off and just eat. Sounds pretty crazy, huh? Just eating? Like a normal person? Spending your energy and efforts on something other than food and exercise worries? I know, it may sound unattainable, but it's possible and I believe it's God's best for you!

VARIETY

We need variety in our diets. Barring food allergies, eating all food groups allows the body to obtain the most diverse nutrient profile. From this, the body is able to take what it needs to function at its best.

In today's culture variety is hard to come by. If we eat mainly processed foods and fast food, those foods tend to be made from a short list of ingredients like wheat, soy, and corn. On the flip side, if we've followed modern fad diet recommendations, we've often eliminated so many food groups that the choices we have left leave us with very little variety in our diets. Either way, avoiding food groups or nutrients over time can lead to deficiencies, low energy, illness, injury, and the like. So instead of thinking about what we can eliminate, let's look at the following list of food types and find the things we can add. Beware, these descriptions are not meant to shame you into eating certain foods, and they certainly aren't a substitute for your own intuition.

Rather, I talk about each food group so that you might realize that all foods have something to offer and can provide benefits to our body. Read these descriptions as more evidence that all foods fit, and you might find what you need to start adding, including those foods you've neglected.

FRUITS & VEGETABLES

Besides providing energy and fiber, fruits and vegetables are rich in micronutrients such as potassium, folate, vitamins A and C, and phytochemicals. There are nutrients and benefits of fruits and veggies that we are STILL discovering. Needless to say, they provide our bodies with a lot of the nutrients they need.

If you think you don't like fruits or vegetables, I'd urge you to reconsider. Do you not like them, or do you just dislike a certain trendy variety, like kale or Brussels sprouts? Further, maybe you haven't tried preparing them with fat or other flavor enhancers. You don't have to like the same produce that the Instagram model does, and you don't have to eat raw and organic only in order to meet your needs. In fact, some nutrients in produce become more available to the body with a little bit of cooking. So, if this is a food group you're lacking, understand that you just need to start small and get creative with how you cook it. With experimentation and persistence, you can find a way to enjoy produce, I promise.

EGGS

Eggs used to get a bad name because of their cholesterol and saturated fat makeup, but we've since found out that dietary cholesterol doesn't raise blood cholesterol and the link between saturated fat and heart disease is a lot less clear than we once thought.[2] What eggs do contain is a inexpensive, natural source of protein and fat, along with B5, selenium, iron, and countless other beneficial vitamins and minerals. Recently, farmers have begun to change the diets of their chickens, resulting in some eggs being a good source of the anti-inflammatory omega-3 fatty acids as well.

MEAT

Red meat from beef, pork, lamb, deer, etc. is another food group that's taken a beating over the years. But we're finding that red meat has a lot of nutrients to offer, especially in its minimally processed form—not to mention all that flavor! Red meat is a rich source of protein, B vitamins—especially B12—iron, zinc, phosphorus, and omega-3 fatty acids, especially when it comes from grass-fed animals. Red meat is definitely a part of a healthy diet, and research is now finding that the correlation between red meat and cardiovascular disease risk is possibly more related to processed meat consumption.[3] So, if you want to, go ahead and enjoy your hamburger and nutrient stores in peace!

FISH

Fish is another excellent source of protein, omega-3 fatty acids, and various vitamins and minerals, including vitamin D, riboflavin, and calcium. Here in the southern Midwest, we don't eat a lot of fish. It's hard to come by with land surrounding us on all sides, and by the time it gets to us it doesn't taste all that great. So, if you have a hard time including fish in your diet, but you feel great and can get those nutrients from another protein source, don't feel ashamed about not eating a lot of fish. However, if you are interested in a relatively tasty and convenient form of fish, I recommend trying canned salmon and using it on salads and pasta or in a salmon patty. You can also buy flash frozen fish at the grocery store and thaw it. Ultimately the decision is up to you, nobody is forcing you to eat fish, but if you want to, and feel led to include it, there's a way.

POULTRY

Like red meat and fish, poultry is a great source of protein, vitamins, and minerals. Lighter meats still contain iron, but in much lower quantities than dark meat and red meat.

DAIRY

Dairy provides us with protein, carbohydrates, fat, and vitamins and minerals, especially calcium, magnesium, and vitamin D. The fat provided in full-fat dairy products is no longer thought to be associated with cardiovascular disease.[4] In fact, some newer research may point to it being beneficial for heart health.[5] Further, nutrients in dairy fat may be beneficial for women trying to conceive [6] and are helpful in early childhood development. Just another instance where man tried to outsmart nature by taking the fat out of dairy and finding out that every food God made is good to eat. Having said that, does that mean eating low fat dairy or dairy substitutes is bad? No, if you prefer it, your body can still use it to nourish you. If you don't tolerate milk, you may be able to tolerate yogurt, cheeses, and lactose free milk. If none of those sit well, I suggest soy milk as a comparable alternative.

WHOLE GRAINS

Whole grains like whole wheat, brown rice, millet, oats, faro, bulgur, quinoa, and barley provide a dense source of energy from carbohydrates, protein, and fat. They're also a great source of fiber, B vitamins, iron, magnesium, selenium, and folate. The last nutrient is so important to fetal development that when we switched to refined flour, the government saw fit to supplement our flour with folic acid (the synthetic form) to ensure the health of our nation's developing babies. Besides, the fiber in whole grains may play an important role in keeping us full for longer and in helping feed the good bacteria in our guts—the bacteria responsible for maintaining health in the digestive tract.

NUTS & SEEDS

Nuts and seeds like almonds, walnuts, macadamia nuts, pistachios, chia, and flax are a great source of beneficial fats, fiber, carbohydrates, protein, and micronutrients like magnesium, vitamin E, and selenium. They taste great in pureed form. I'm sure many of you have met one of my best friends—nut butter! You can snack on these guys, roast them and add them to recipes, blend them into smoothies, add them to your cereal—the possibilities are endless.

LEGUMES

Legumes include every variety of beans: black, pinto, kidney, lima, navy, garbanzo, soy, as well as lentils and peanuts. They provide the best source of plant protein, along with fiber, vitamins, and minerals. They're relatively inexpensive, last a long time, and are easy to flavor, as they absorb the taste of whatever they're cooked with!

FUN FOODS

Lest you think I was pulling a fast one on you, enter the fun foods category. These are the foods that don't necessarily fit into just one of the above food groups. It's things like chips, sweets, candy, soda, alcohol, and refined grains. It's the food that you might be tempted to cut out completely because you don't see it listed above. But the truth is, most of these foods are made from one or more of the above food groups. Our bodies certainly know how to digest and use mixed foods and processed foods. Likewise, all food is broken down into the same tiny components, sugar, fat, protein, and micronutrients and is then used by the body accordingly. Anything that doesn't belong gets filtered out by the liver and kidneys, and thus food does not defile us! However, being stressed out about the food we eat does cause the systems of the body to not function as well as they should, which may cause more damage than any one food. So, here's to food freedom, less stress, and enjoying fun foods!

Why did I just give you a run down on every single food group? Was it to make you feel guilty for not eating the foods in those groups? No. Rather, I hope that by reading this you realize that every food has something to offer that benefits our bodies. We don't need to like every food or even eat every food within those groups. But the more open we are to trying new foods and eating from most, if not all, food groups, the less energy we'll have to spend planning and worrying about our every meal, the more we can be thankful for the gift of food, and the better we'll be able to supply our bodies with what they need.

Maybe something in this chapter stuck out to you as new information. Maybe you feel led to start including more foods from a certain group in your diet. Or maybe you feel led to add a little bit more balance at meal time. I'd encourage you to give that decision to God, ask Him to help you fuel your body, and to have grace for yourself when that's not always how it goes. Above all, remember that if you make Him the manager of your life, He has the power to break all bondage to food and He's a good leader, one who is more than able and willing to care for your living body. You are loved, you are redeemed, and you are worth it to Him.

No matter what food you eat or don't eat, no matter what you can afford or not afford, He will be faithful to care for you and bless you, if you'll let Him in, if you'll stop following the world's misplaced rules, stop striving for your own will and instead start leaning on Him, trusting in His goodness, and believing you are who He says you are! That, my friends is the source of real health and a far weightier thing to savor than any superfood, nutrient, or "perfectly" balanced diet.

REFLECTION QUESTIONS

1. How do you feel about reading nutrition information at this point in the book? Do you feel differently about nutrition recommendations or do they still make you anxious? If so, pray about this and go back to focusing on God's grace and making peace with food.

2. What behaviors, if any, is God leading you to implement? It may be as simple as eating regularly or adding carbohydrates into your day.

3. Have you made God the manager of your life? Do you believe that just as he raised a dead body from the dead, He is capable of managing a living body?

4. Is there anything you learned about in this chapter that made you feel more at ease around food? Is there any food you're inspired to try?

Chapter 15

LIVING FREE IN A CULTURE OF BONDAGE

"Beloved friends, what should be our proper response to God's marvelous mercies? I encourage you to surrender yourselves to God to be his sacred, living sacrifices. And live in holiness, experiencing all that delights his heart. For this becomes your genuine expression of worship. Stop imitating the ideals and opinions of the culture around you, but be inwardly transformed by the Holy Spirit through a total reformation of how you think. This will empower you to discern God's will as you live a beautiful life, satisfying and perfect in his eyes."

ROMANS 12:1-2 TPT

NOW THAT YOU KNOW

Now that you know the truth, what will you do? I could tell you what I did when I discovered it, but first let's answer the question: what truth have we discovered? The truth that our worth is far greater than our appearance. The truth that grace has already made us wholly accepted, wholly loved, and wholly redeemed. The truth that God wants to bless us with health, but that He needs our hearts in order to do this. The truth that we are already a new creation in Christ, that we can stop striving to earn His love and the acceptance of others, and we can stop slaving away towards an unrealistic standard of perfection that already exists in Christ. The truth that all foods fit, and that food can't save us or defile us. The truth that movement can be enjoyable. The truth that we can trust the body God gave us, and we no longer need to micromanage it. The truth that God is a far better manager of our lives than we are, and only He has the power to break the bondage of food, exercise, and body image concerns over our lives. The truth that only He can give real, vibrant health and He is faithful to do it.

That truth. Now that you know it, you won't be the same. It will be hard to listen to the lies of the enemy as they permeate every part of our culture. It will be hard to watch someone you love struggle with the same things you once did and feel like they just aren't seeing reason. At least that's how it was for me.

And if I'm being honest, I became a little angry for a time, judgmental for a time, and lonely for a time. I've been rejected, misunderstood, and persecuted for sharing these truths. And we're just talking about food! That doesn't account for the persecution that the message of radical grace seems to bring from both outside and inside the church. After a little while, God showed me that it was not my job to judge others, or even correct them, every time they said something contrary to what I'd learned. No, my job (maybe our job) as a Christian, is to love people the way God has loved us, unconditionally. We must offer grace in extravagant doses, just as we have been offered it. We must love people first and not judge them because we too were once blind, and in certain areas, still are in certain areas. I think we'll find there will be more opportunities to speak truth into other's lives if we will just love them where they are and live out what we believe.

Love first, always offer grace, share truth in love when the opportunity is right, and leave your opinions for last, or just leave them completely out. May we be known for our love and not our opinions. When we do this, the freedom we enjoy will be a light to people around us and not a stumbling block.

GUARD YOUR HEART

As you go out into the world of diets, food rules, and one million different idols. As you enter into the realm of striving and condemnation, remember that you still live in a fallen world, one where the enemy is very real and present, and one where people are still very lost. The Bible warns us to guard our hearts above all else, and so we should. But what does this look like? We can't completely shut ourselves off from the lost, that's not what Jesus did, and we're not going to be known for loving others while living like hermits. Matthew 6:22 tells us that the eye is the lamp of the body, that when our eye is good, our whole bodies will be full of light. In other words, what we see, what we think on, and what we imagine impacts us. We can guard our hearts by being careful with the information that we consume and the things that we look at.

Practically, this might mean unfollowing social media accounts that promote strict food rules, over exercising, or anything else that speaks against the truth you believe, or your values. It may mean spending more time around people that lift you up and a little less around those that don't. It may also mean being selective with who you open up to about your food and body image beliefs or struggles. If you're uncertain of the grace or advice someone will or won't offer you, then seek out someone who will support you in grace and truth. There is a large community of Christians who promote food freedom. You can find resources like podcasts, blogs, and books to connect with. You may also find new, non-diet social media accounts to follow.

Once we've cleaned out the junk, it's imperative that we continually fill our hearts with the pure and perfect truth. The first, and primary source, is the Bible. Go to the Word and read in search of Jesus, seeking to know Him, and to know God's character. Look for His grace, provision, and promises. If your experience is anything like mine, once you have a revelation of God's great grace and a realization that accusations and condemnation come from the enemy, the Bible will come alive. Passages that never made much sense will finally be clear. And when you don't understand a passage, ask the Holy Spirit to teach you, and He will. Continue to ask God for more of His Holy Spirit, more guidance, and more power to live separate in a world full of bondage.

Finally, hold on to the truth that you've heard and be set free. Do not conform to the patterns of our world, but daily renew your mind with the truth and you will be transformed, from the inside out.

REFLECTION QUESTIONS

1. Of all the truths mentioned at the beginning of this chapter, which has been most transforming and freeing for you?

2. How does this change your view of the culture at large and even the practices of some of the people in your life? How can you love them where they are?

3. What filters do you need to put in place in your life in order to guard your heart well?

4. How can you hold onto the truth daily? Check out the resources section. What are some resources you want to investigate?

HELPFUL RESOURCES

1. *Caroline Williams* **yoga youtube** offers free online yoga practices that center around scripture and drawing nearer to Christ. She also has a website and a group membership called *the Abbey.*

2. *Eating with Grace* **podcast,** hosted by Christine Hebert, MS, RD, CDN, is a faith focused podcast exploring the concepts of intuitive eating, body acceptance, and worth in Christ.

3. *Finding Balance,* a Christ-centered 501(c)(3) nonprofit, is "dedicated to helping people find freedom from eating issues" and operates a website and support network that holds online group sessions for disordered eating and eating disorder recovery among more.

4. **The book** *Intuitive Eating* by Evelyn Tribole M.S. R.D. and Elyse Resch M.S. R.D. F.A.D.A. explains the principles of intuitive eating, the science behind them, and how to put them into practice.

5. **The** *NEDA helpline* is run by the National Eating Disorders Association and offers support, resources and treatment options for yourself and/or a loved one. Visit https://www.nationaleatingdisorders.org/help-

support/contact-helpline for contact information and hours of operation.

6. **The *Revelation Wellness* podcast** is a faith focused podcast that provides wellness and fitness meditations, and encouragement for your workout.

WORKS CITED

CHAPTER 1

1. Reba-Harreleson, L., Holle, A. V., Hamer, R. M., Swann, R., Reyes, M. L., & Bulik, C. M. (2009). Patterns and Prevalence of Disordered Eating and Weight Control Behaviors in Women Ages 25–45. Eating and Weight Disorders : EWD, 14(4), e190–e198.

2. Hudson, J. I., Hiripi, E., Pope, H. G., & Kessler, R. C. (2007). The Prevalence and Correlates of Eating Disorders in the National Comorbidity Survey Replication. Biological Psychiatry, 61(3), 348–358. http://doi.org/10.1016/j.biopsych.2006.03.040

3. Le Grange, D., Swanson, S. A., Crow, S. J., & Merikangas, K. R. (2012). Eating disorder not otherwise specified presentation in the US population. The International Journal of Eating Disorders, 45(5), 711–718. http://doi.org/10.1002/eat.22006

CHAPTER 2

1. W. Gray, S., & J. Fernandez, S. (1989). Effects of visuo-motor behavior rehearsal with videotaped modeling on basketball shooting performance.

2. Elsenbruch, S. (2011). Abdominal pain in Irritable Bowel Syndrome: A review of putative psychlogical, neural and neuro-immune mechanisms. Brain, Behavior, and Immunity, 25(3), 386-394.

3. Beuchner, F. (1973). *Wishful Thinking: A Theological ABC*. New York, NY: Harper & Row.

CHAPTER 3

1. Condemn [Def. 1]. (n.d.). *Merriam-Webster Online*. In Merriam-Webster. Retrieved July 1, 2018, from http://www.merriam-webster.com/dictionary/condemn

CHAPTER 5

1. Keys, A., et al. (2014). "Indices of relative weight and obesity*." International Journal of Epidemiology 43(3): 655-665.

2. Rey-López, J. P., et al. (2014). "The prevalence of metabolically healthy obesity: a systematic review and critical evaluation of the definitions used." Obesity Reviews 15(10): 781-790.

3. Raghupathi, W., & Raghupathi, V. (2018). An Empirical Study of Chronic Diseases in the United States: A Visual Analytics Approach to Public Health. *International Journal of Environmental Research and Public Health, 15*(3), 431. doi: 10.3390/ijerph15030431

4. Bacon, L., & Aphramor, L. (2011). Weight Science: Evaluating the Evidence for a Paradigm Shift. Nutrition Journal, 10(1), 9. doi: 10.1186/1475-2891-10-9

5. Matheson, E. M., King, D. E., & Everett, C. J. (2012). Healthy lifestyle habits and mortality in overweight and obese individuals. J Am Board Fam Med, 25(1), 9-15. doi: 10.3122/jabfm.2012.01.110164

CHAPTER 7

1. Bacon, L., & Aphramor, L. (2011). Weight Science: Evaluating the Evidence for a Paradigm Shift. Nutrition Journal, 10(1), 9. doi: 10.1186/1475-2891-10-9

2. Schwingshackl, L., Schwedhelm, C., Hoffmann, G., Lampousi, A.-M., Knüppel, S., Iqbal, K., . . . Boeing, H. (2017). Food groups and risk of all-cause mortality: a systematic review and meta-analysis of prospective studies. The American Journal of Clinical Nutrition, 105(6), 1462-1473. doi: 10.3945/ajcn.117.153148

CHAPTER 8

1. Dickerhoof, C.E. and Miller, D. [Funny or Die]. (2017). *This is why eating healthy is hard time traveling dietitian.* Retrieved from https://www.funnyordie.com/2017/7/26/17722222/this-is-why-eating-healthy-is-hard-time-travel-dietician

2. Ziauddeen, H., & Fletcher, P. C. (2013). Is food addiction a valid and useful concept? Obesity Reviews, 14(1), 19-28. doi: 10.1111/j.1467-789X.2012.01046.

CHAPTER 9

1. Simmons, B. (2018). 2 Timothy. The Passion Translation New Testament with Psalms, Proverbs and Song of Songs, Second Edition. (pp 603 footnote a). Broadstreet Publishing.

2. 1 Timothy 1:7, Darby Bible Translation

3. Mann, T. et al. (2007).Medicare's search for effective obesity treatments: Diets are not the answer. American Psychologist, 62(3): 220-233.
    Field, A,E. et al (2003). Relation Between Dieting and Weight Change Among Preadolescents and Adolescents. Pediatrics,112:900-906. [Free Full Texthttp://pediatrics.aappublications.org/content/112/4/900.long]

Haines, J. & Neumark-Sztainer D (2006). Prevention of obesity and eating disorders: a consideration of shared risk factors. Health Education Research, 21(6):770–782. [Free Full Texthttp://her.oxfordjournals.org/content/21/6/770.long]

Neumark-Sztainer, D. et al (2006). Obesity, disordered eating, and eating disorders in a longitudinal study of adolescents: how do dieters fare five years later? J Am Diet Assoc,106(4):559-568.

Patton, G. C., et al. (1999). Onset of adolescent eating disorders: population based cohort study over 3 years. British Medical Journal, 318:765-768. [Free Full Text http://www.bmj.com/content/318/7186/765?view=long&pmid=10082698].

Pietiläinen, K.H. et al. (2011). Does dieting make you fat? A twin study. International Journal of Obesity, | doi:10.1038/ijo.2011.160

Saarni, S. E. et al (2006). Weight cycling of athletes and subsequent weight gain in middleage. International J Obesity, 30: 1639–1644. [Free full text at http://bit.ly/yvfnhE]

Tribole E. & Resch E. (2012-in press). Intuitive Eating (3rd edition). St.Martin's Press: NY,NY.

CHAPTER 10:

1. Breit, S., Kupferberg, A., Rogler, G., & Hasler, G. (2018). Vagus Nerve as Modulator of the Brain–Gut Axis in Psychiatric and Inflammatory Disorders. Frontiers in Psychiatry, 9, 44. doi: 10.3389/fpsyt.2018.00044

CHAPTER 11:

1. Hallberg, L., Björn-Rasmussen, E., Rossander, L., & Suwanik, R. (1977). Iron absorption from Southeast Asian diets. II. Role of various factors that might explain low absorption. *The American Journal of Clinical Nutrition, 30*(4), 539-548. doi: 10.1093/ajcn/30.4.539

2. Lam, J. (2015). Picky Eating in Children. Frontiers in Pediatrics, 3, 41. doi: 10.3389/fped.2015.00041

CHAPTER 12:

1. Ambrose, K. R., & Golightly, Y. M. (2015). Physical exercise as non-pharmacological treatment of chronic pain: Why and when. Best practice & research. Clinical rheumatology, 29(1), 120-130. doi: 10.1016/j.berh.2015.04.022

2. Physical Activity. (2018, February 13). Retrieved from https://www.cdc.gov/physicalactivity/basics/pa-health/index.htm

3. Eusebeia – New Testament Greek Lexicon – New American Standard. (n.d.) Retrieved from https://www.biblestudytools.com/lexicons/greek/nas/eusebeia.html

CHAPTER 14:

1. Davis, C. M. (1939). Results of the self-selection of diets by young children. Canadian Medical Association Journal, 41(3), 257-261.

2. Blesso, C. N., & Fernandez, M. L. (2018). Dietary Cholesterol, Serum Lipids, and Heart Disease: Are Eggs Working for or Against You? Nutrients, 10(4), 426. doi: 10.3390/nu10040426

3. Micha, R., Wallace, S. K., & Mozaffarian, D. (2010). Red and processed meat consumption and risk of incident coronary heart disease, stroke, and diabetes: A systematic review and meta-analysis. Circulation, 121(21), 2271-2283. doi: 10.1161/CIRCULATIONAHA.109.924977

4. Lordan, R., Tsoupras, A., Mitra, B., & Zabetakis, I. (2018). Dairy Fats and Cardiovascular Disease: Do We Really Need to Be Concerned? Foods, 7(3), 29. doi: 10.3390/foods7030029

5. de Oliveira Otto, M. C., Lemaitre, R. N., Song, X., King, I. B., Siscovick, D. S., & Mozaffarian, D. (2018). Serial measures of circulating biomarkers of dairy fat and total and cause-specific mortality in older adults: the Cardiovascular Health Study. The American Journal of Clinical Nutrition, 108(3), 476-484. doi: 10.1093/ajcn/nqy117

6. Chavarro, J. E., Rich-Edwards, J. W., Rosner, B., & Willett, W. C. (2007). A prospective study of dairy foods intake and anovulatory infertility. Human Reproduction, 22(5), 1340-1347. doi: 10.1093/humrep/dem019

ACKNOWLEDGEMENTS

Thanks to my husband for giving me grace in the most tangible ways, every single day. Thank you to my parents for modeling the Father's love and always encouraging me to be who God called me to be. Thanks to my clients who teach me more than I teach them. Thank you to all the amazing colleagues, friends, and family who have helped me share this message. But thanks, above all, to my beautiful savior, who never stops saving me, never stops loving me, and never stops pouring out his overflowing grace for me.

ABOUT THE AUTHOR

Aubrey Golbek, MS, RDN lives in Tulsa, OK with her husband and children. She is a writer, dietitian, and mom with a passion for God's word and food freedom. Aubrey owns Grace Fueled Nutrition, a private nutrition counseling practice. She focuses on disordered eating, sports nutrition, and women's wellness.

You can read more at www.gracefueled.com

Made in the USA
Coppell, TX
24 March 2021

52236099R00132